Contents

KT-226-624

Introduction

Trying to follow a healthy diet when money is tight isn't easy, but it can be done, especially with the help of this collection of 150 tried and tested recipes brought to you by BBC *Good Food* magazine. We believe that good health starts with good food and a diet that is balanced in all the essential nutrients, incorporates fruit, vegetables, lean protein, healthy fats and unrefined carbohydrates and minimises processed foods.

The following recipes, all with nutritional breakdowns per serving, have been chosen according to their health-giving ingredients, and steer away from faddy foods and luxuries, to ensure that you can eat well all week without breaking the bank. These recipes will nourish you across every mealtime from breakfast to supper whether you are a meat eater or vegetarian.

There are also bakes and desserts that have had healthy makeovers, but be aware that although healthier than their original, they are intended as an occasional treat.

When selecting recipes from this book aim to eat at least 5 portions of vegetables and fruit a day, with the emphasis on vegetables to keep natural sugars to a minimum. The secret is to eat the rainbow, a variety with different colours, to provide your body with a range of nutrients and protective antioxidants. A tip for making the most of your budget is to eat fruit and veg in season, when they are at their peak and cheapest. And don't forget that beans and pulses, juices and dried, canned and frozen fruit and veg all contribute towards your 5 a day.

When it comes to meat it is better to spend more but eat less to ensure you can afford the healthier cuts, so don't dismiss the thought of eating meat-free-meals a couple of times a week even if you are not a vegetarian. And aim to eat white and oily fish at least once a week, too.

Here are some other helpful money-saving tips
- Love your leftovers and eat them for lunch the following day.
- Check your fridge at the end of the week and make use of odds and ends in soups, omelettes and rice dishes.
- Make good use of your freezer as you can save across the board in most frozen food categories.
- Keep a check on your store cupboard. If you have bought a new ingredient such as tahini or red curry paste, make sure you don't waste the rest of the jar.
- Write a shopping list and stick to it.
- Try trading down when it come to brands. According to Money Saving Expert you can save 30 per cent off your shopping bill this way and you probably won't even notice the difference on ingredients such as canned tomatoes.

We hope that this book will give you plenty of inspiration to eat well, and within budget, across the seasons. It isn't how much you spend on the ingredients, but what you do with them that makes the most delicious meals and these recipes, all with colour photos, will show you how.

Sara

Sara Buenfeld

good food eat well

CHEAP & HEALTHY

EDITOR
Sara Buenfeld

BOOKS

10 9 8 7 6 5 4 3 2 1

BBC Books, an imprint of Ebury Publishing
20 Vauxhall Bridge Road,
London SW1V 2SA

BBC Books is part of the Penguin Random House group of companies whose addresses can be found at global.penguinrandomhouse.com

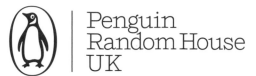

Photographs © BBC Magazines 2016
Recipes © BBC Worldwide 2016
Book design © Woodlands Books Ltd 2016
All recipes contained in this book first appeared in BBC Good Food magazine.

First published by BBC Books in 2016

www.eburypublishing.co.uk

A CIP catalogue record for this book is available from the British Library

ISBN 9781785940736

Printed and bound in Germany by Mohn Media GmbH

Project editor: Charlotte Macdonald
Design: Interstate Creative Partners Ltd and Kathryn Gammon
Cover Design: Interstate Creative Partners Ltd
Production: Alex Goddard
Picture Researcher: Gabby Harrington

Notes & Conversion Tables

NOTES ON THE RECIPES
- Eggs are large in the UK and Australia and extra large in America unless stated.
- Wash fresh produce before preparation.
- Recipes contain nutritional analyses for 'sugar', which means the total sugar content including all natural sugars in the ingredients, unless otherwise stated.

APPROXIMATE WEIGHT CONVERSIONS
- All the recipes in this book list both metric and imperial measurements. Conversions are approximate and have been rounded up or down. Follow one set of measurements only; do not mix the two.
- Cup measurements, which are used in Australia and America, have not been listed here as they vary from ingredient to ingredient. Kitchen scales should be used to measure dry/solid ingredients.

Good Food is concerned about sustainable sourcing and animal welfare. Where possible, humanely reared meats, sustainably caught fish (see fishonline.org for further information from the Marine Conservation Society) and free-range chickens and eggs are used when recipes are originally tested.

OVEN TEMPERATURES

GAS	°C	°C FAN	°F	OVEN TEMP.
¼	110	90	225	Very cool
½	120	100	250	Very cool
1	140	120	275	Cool or slow
2	150	130	300	Cool or slow
3	160	140	325	Warm
4	180	160	350	Moderate
5	190	170	375	Moderately hot
6	200	180	400	Fairly hot
7	220	200	425	Hot
8	230	210	450	Very hot
9	240	220	475	Very hot

SPOON MEASURES
Spoon measurements are level unless otherwise specified.
- 1 teaspoon (tsp) = 5ml
- 1 tablespoon (tbsp) = 15ml
- 1 Australian tablespoon = 20ml
(cooks in Australia should measure 3 teaspoons where 1 tablespoon is specified in a recipe)

APPROXIMATE LIQUID CONVERSIONS

Metric	Imperial	AUS	US
50ml	2fl oz	¼ cup	¼ cup
125ml	4fl oz	½ cup	½ cup
175ml	6fl oz	¾ cup	¾ cup
225ml	8fl oz	1 cup	1 cup
300ml	10fl oz/½ pint	½ pint	1¼ cups
450ml	16fl oz	2 cups	2 cups/1 pint
600ml	20fl oz/1 pint	1 pint	2½ cups
1 litre	35fl oz/1¾ pints	1¾ pints	1 quart

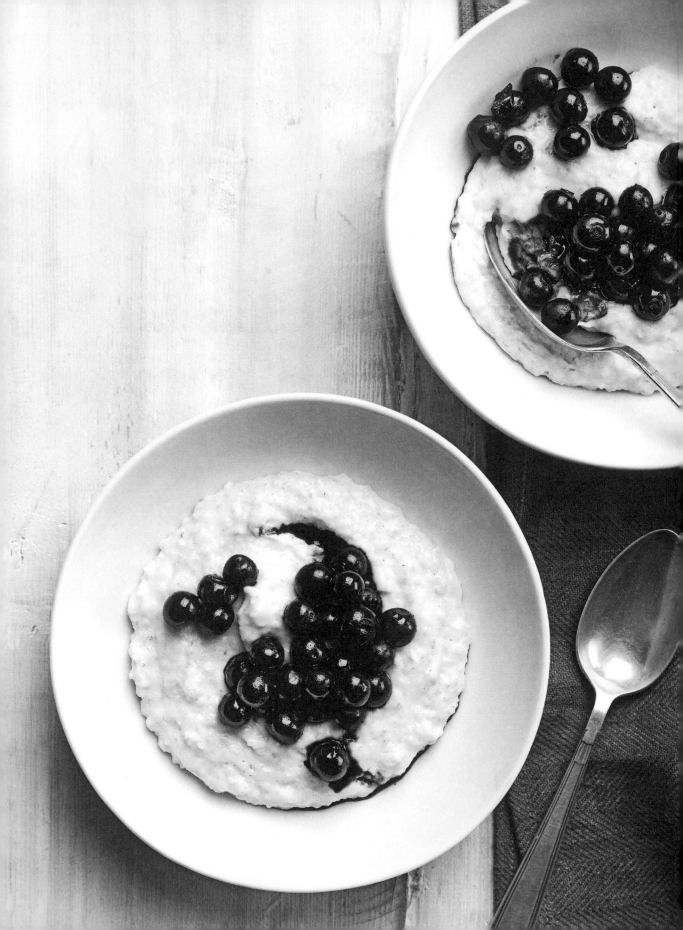

Chapter 1:

BREAKFAST, BRUNCH & SMOOTHIES

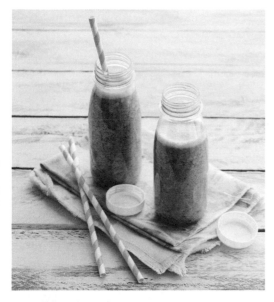
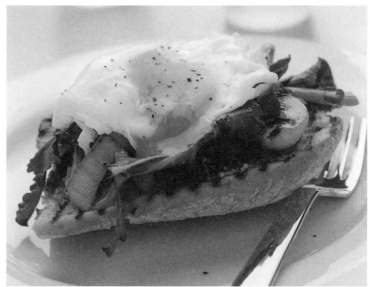
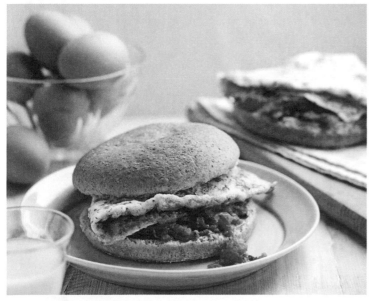
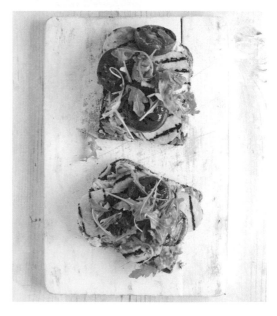

Fruit & Nut Breakfast Bowl

Top cheap and healthy porridge with Greek yogurt, fresh oranges and a sprinkling of dried fruit, nuts and seeds for a filling, vitamin-C-rich start to your day.

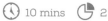 10 mins   2

- 6 tbsp porridge oats
- 2 oranges
- just under half a 200ml tub 0% fat Greek-style yogur
- 60g pot raisins, nuts, goji berries and seeds

1 Put the oats in a non-stick pan with 400ml water and cook over the heat, stirring occasionally, for about 2 mins until thickened.
2 Meanwhile, cut the peel and pith from the oranges then slice them in half, cutting down either side as closely as you can to where the stalk would be – this will remove quite a tough section of the membrane. Now just chop the oranges.
3 Pour the porridge into bowls, spoon on the yogurt then pile on the oranges and dried fruit, nut and seed mixture.

PER SERVING 316 kcals, fat 11g, saturates 1g, carbs 35g, sugars 18g, fibre 7g, protein 15g, salt 0.1g

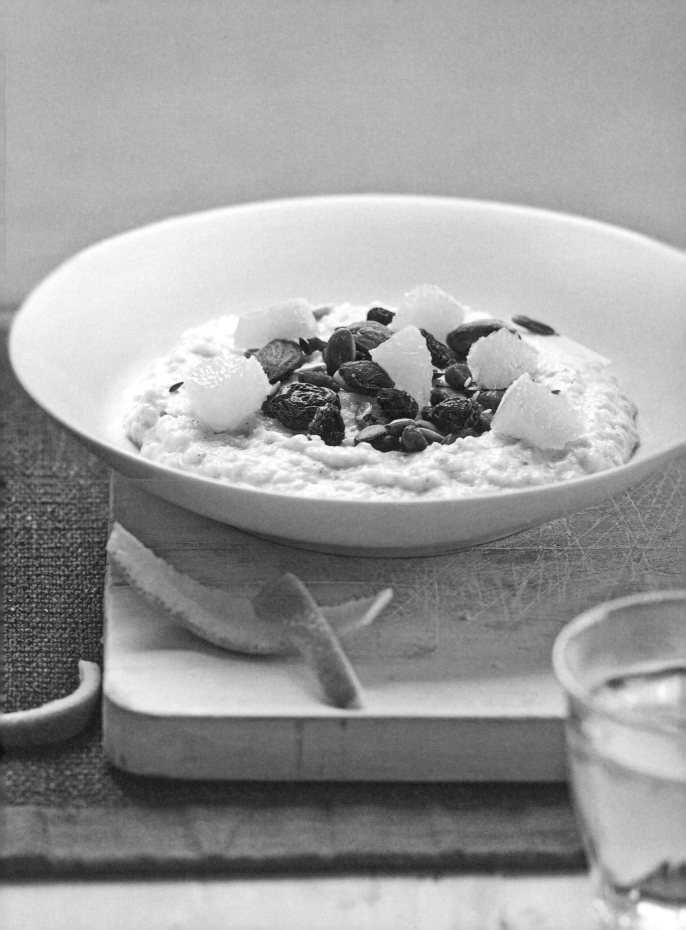

Porridge with Blueberry Compote

Not just a slow-releasing source of energy, oats are high in fibre and will help to control your cholesterol, too. Frozen blueberries are much cheaper than fresh and so are perfect here.

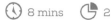 8 mins   2

- 6 tbsp porridge oats
- just under ½ a 200ml tub 0%-fat Greek-style yogurt
- 175g/6oz frozen blueberries
- 1 tsp honey (optional)

1 Put the oats in a non-stick pan with 400ml water and cook over the heat, stirring occasionally, for about 2 mins until thickened. Remove from the heat and add a third of the yogurt.
2 Meanwhile, tip the blueberries into a pan with 1 tbsp water and the honey, if using, and gently poach until the blueberries have thawed and they are tender, but still holding their shape.
3 Spoon the porridge into bowls, top with the remaining yogurt and spoon over the blueberries.

PER SERVING 168 kcals, fat 2g, saturates 1g, carbs 24g, sugars 9g, fibre 5g, protein 9g, salt none

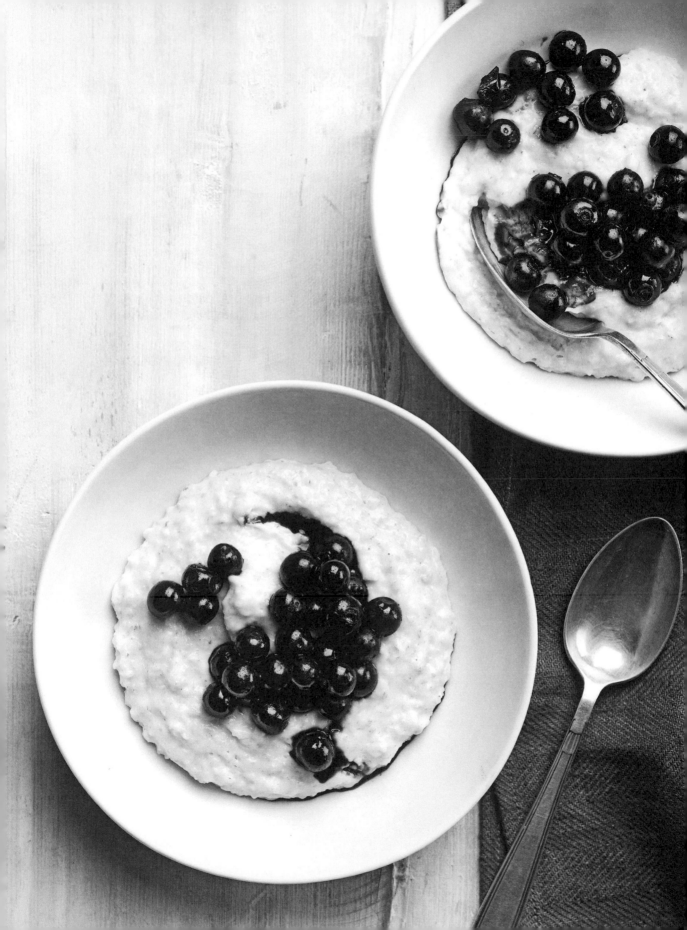

Pear & Blueberry Bircher

If you don't have fresh or frozen blueberries, a heaped tablespoon of raisins will count as 1 of your 5 a day instead. Add them with the oats so they have time to plump up in the yogurt.

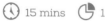 15 mins 1

- 1 firm but ripe pear, no need to peel
- 2 tbsp oats
- 150g pot 0% fat bio yogurt
- 3 tbsp skimmed milk, plus a bit extra
- 1 tbsp pumpkin seeds
- 2 handfuls blueberries, fresh or just thawed if frozen

1 Grate the pear into a bowl and add the oats, half the yogurt and milk with most of the seeds. Leave for about 5-10 mins then check the consistency and dilute with a little more milk or water if it is too thick for you. Spoon on the remaining yogurt, pile on the berries and remaining seeds and serve.

PER SERVING 415 kcals, fat 9.7g, saturates 1.7g, carbs 56.6g, sugars 35.8g, fibre 10.6g, protein 20g, salt 0.3g

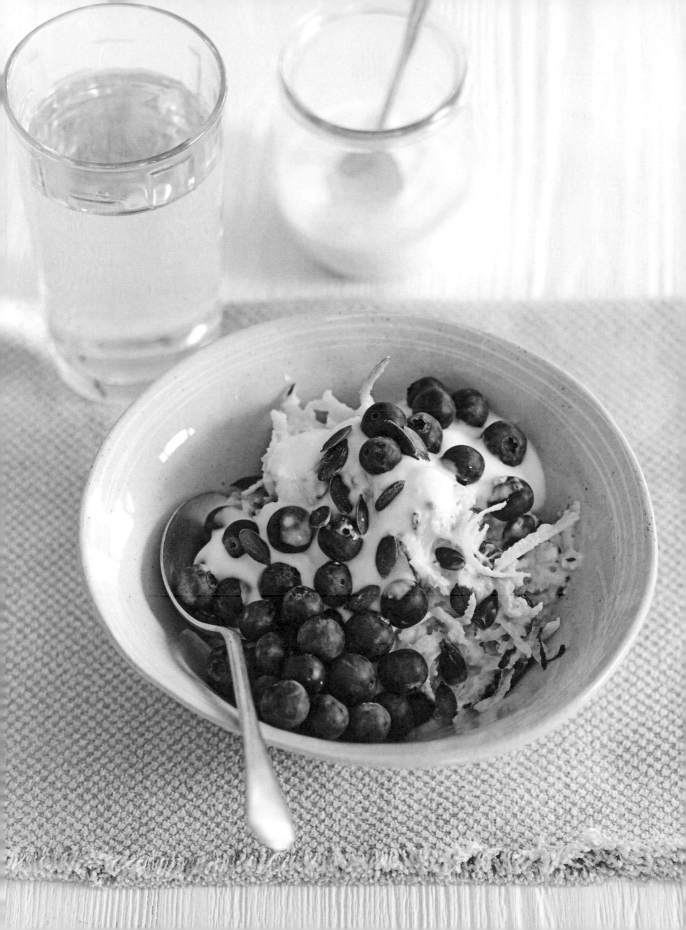

Apricot, Ginger & Grapefruit Compote

This is really zingy and refreshing, delicious with probiotic yogurt or porridge.

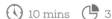 10 mins 3

- 300g can breakfast apricots
- 1 tsp finely grated fresh ginger
- 2 pink grapefruits, peeled and cut into segments
- ½ handful sunflower seeds or flaked almonds to serve (optional)

1 Tip the apricots and their juice into a bowl, add the ginger then blitz half the mixture with a stick blender to puree it and turn the juice into more of a sauce. Stir in the grapefruit segments and chill until ready to serve.
2 Use to top porridge or yogurt, or scatter with seeds or nuts for some crunch, if you like.

PER SERVING 171 kcals, fat 3g, saturates 1g, carbs 42g, sugars 17g, fibre 2g, protein 4g, salt 0.4g

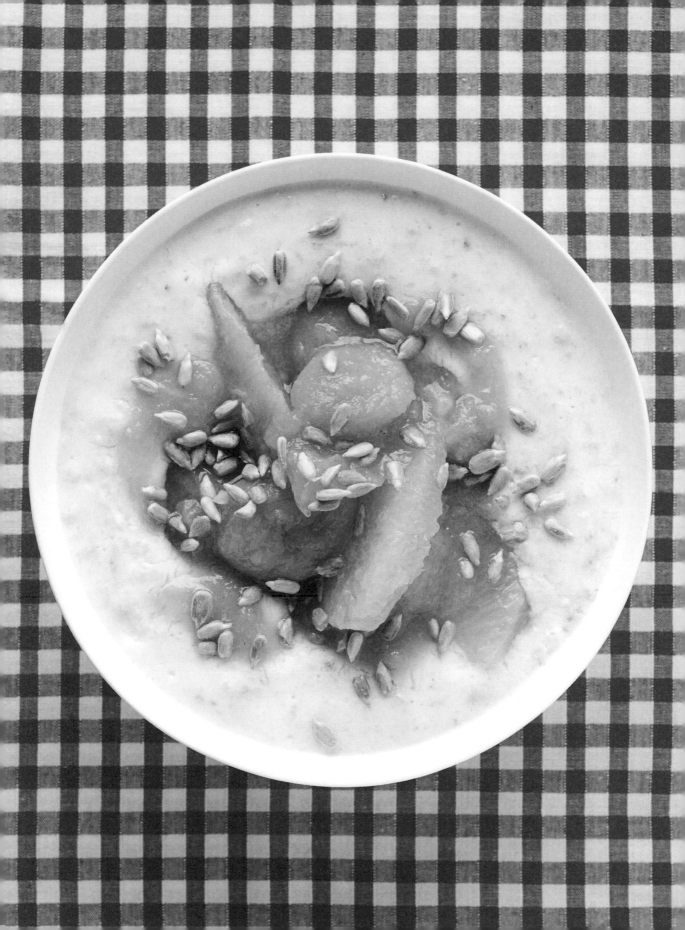

Ricotta Pancakes with Winter Compote

These light and fluffy pancakes make a great weekend brunch served with a compote of apples, dates, pears and cinnamon. For an easy morning, they can be made ahead.

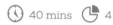 40 mins · 4

- 2 apples, peeled, cored and cut into wedges
- 2 pears, peeled, cored and cut into chunks
- 4 dates, stoned and chopped
- 1 cinnamon stick or ¼ tsp ground
- 3 oranges, juice of 1 and 2 segmented
- 140g/5oz 0% fat Greek yogurt
- 1 tsp vanilla extract
- 140g/5oz plain flour
- 1 tsp baking powder
- 2 large eggs, separated
- 150ml/¼ pint skimmed milk
- 175g/6oz ricotta
- 1 tbsp rapeseed or vegetable oil

1 Cook the apples, pears, dates, cinnamon and orange juice in a saucepan with 1 tbsp of water on a low heat for 15-20 mins until the fruit is soft and juices have thickened. In a small bowl, mix the yogurt with the vanilla. Set aside.

2 Meanwhile, sift the flour and baking powder into a bowl, and whisk the egg yolks, milk and ricotta in a jug until smooth. In another bowl, beat the egg whites until stiff peaks form.

3 Pour the ricotta mix into the flour, whisking together briefly. Gently fold in the egg whites in two batches.

4 Heat a little of the oil in a large, non-stick frying pan. Dollop in a spoonful of the pancake mixture – you're looking to make about 12 pancakes from the batter. Fry for 1-2 mins on each side until puffed up and cooked through. Pile up on a plate with some foil placed loosely on top to keep them warm. Repeat to use up all the batter.

5 Stir the orange segments through the compote and warm through. Serve the pancakes with a spoonful of compote and a dollop of the vanilla yogurt.

PER SERVING 370 kcals, fat 11g, saturates 4g, carbs 53g, sugars 27g, fibre 6g, protein 15g, salt 0.6g

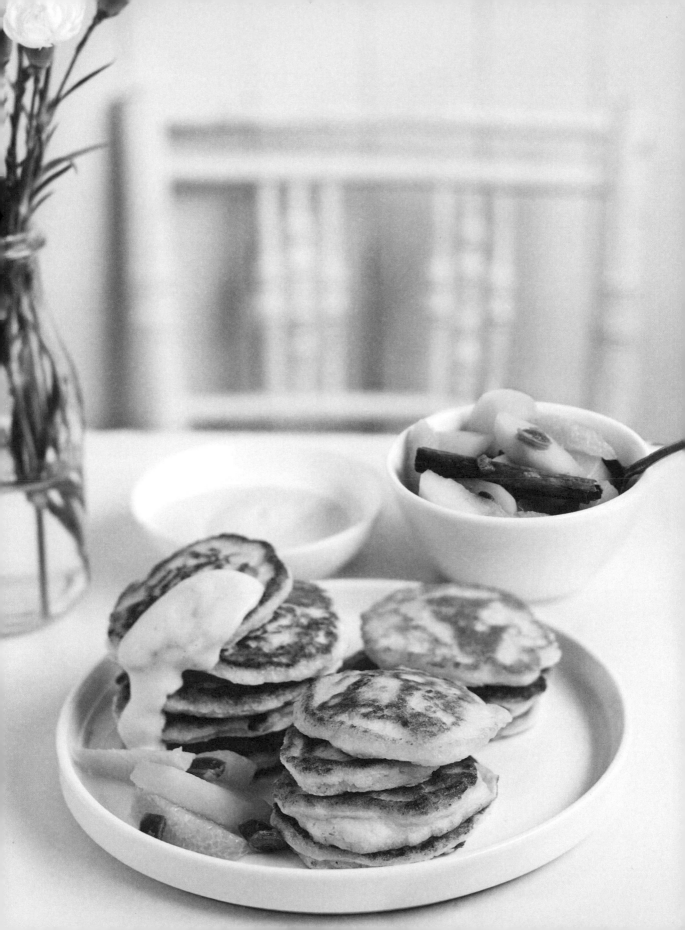

Cinnamon & Almond Granola

If you want a dairy-free oat milk with this, blitz 200g oats in a processor with 500ml water then strain through muslin to get a milk the consistency of single cream.

🕐 1 hour 40 mins   🥧 4

- juice 2 oranges (150ml/¼ pint juice), plus zest of ½
- 200g/7oz jumbo oats
- 1 tsp ground cinnamon
- 2 tbsp freeze-dried strawberries, or raspberries or sultanas
- 25g/1oz toasted flaked almonds
- 25g/1oz mixed seeds (such as sunflower, pumpkin, sesame and linseed)
- dairy or oat milk, to serve
- orange segments and mint leaves (optional)

1 Heat oven to 200C/180C fan/gas 6 and line a baking tray with baking parchment. Put the orange juice in a medium saucepan and bring to the boil. Boil rapidly for 5 mins or until the liquid has reduced by half, stirring occasionally

2 Mix the oats with the orange zest and cinnamon. Remove the pan from the heat and stir the oat mixture into the juice. Spread over the lined tray in a thin layer and bake for 10-15 mins or until lightly browned and crisp, turning the oats every few mins. Leave to cool on the tray.

3 Once cool, mix the oats with your choice of dried fruit, the flaked almonds and seeds. This can be kept in a sealed jar for up to one week. To serve, spoon the granola into bowls, pour over the milk and top with the orange segments and mint leaves, if you like.

PER SERVING 282 kcals, fat 10g, saturates 1g, carbs 32g, sugars 4g, fibre 7g, protein 12g, salt none

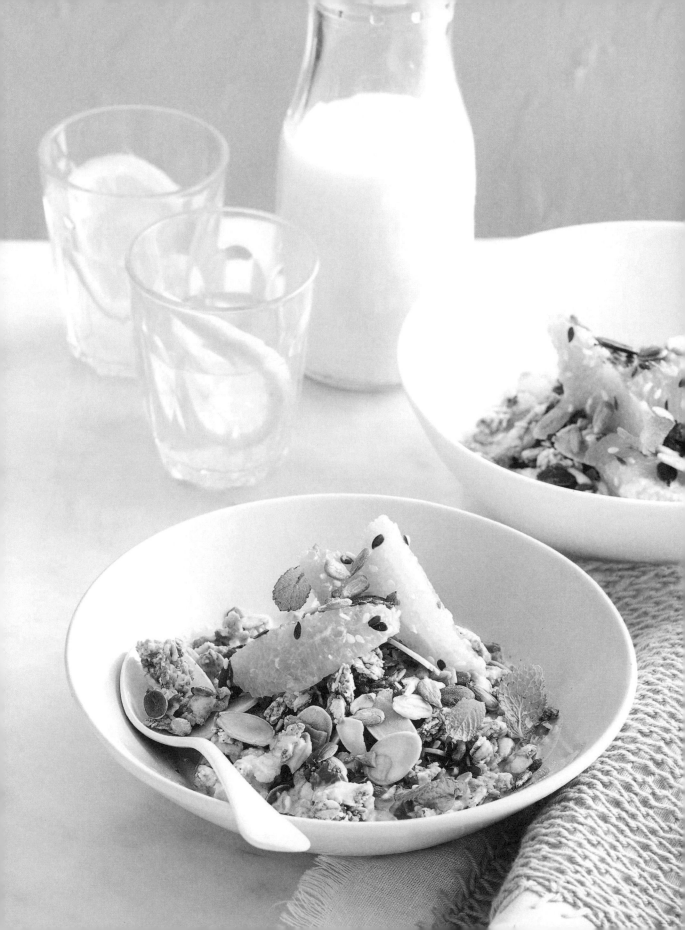

Clementine & Honey Couscous

Although not usually served for breakfast, nuts, clementines, honey and cinnamon make couscous a perfect start to your day. A great way to use any ends of couscous packs, too.

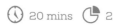 20 mins 2

- 50g/2oz shelled nuts, use a mixture or one type, like almonds, walnuts or pistachios
- 140g/15oz couscous
- a few generous pinches ground cinnamon
- 4 clementines
- 1 tsp butter
- 1 tbsp clear honey, plus extra to serve
- 140g/5oz fresh or frozen raspberries
- reduced-fat Greek yogurt, to serve

1 Heat oven to 200C/180C fan/gas 6. Spread the nuts over a baking sheet and toast for 5-8 mins.
2 Meanwhile, put the couscous and cinnamon into a large bowl. Finely grate the zest from 1 clementine, then squeeze their juice into a pan with the zest. Add the butter, honey and 100ml water and bring to the boil. Pour this over the couscous, cover with cling film, then leave to absorb for 10 mins.
3 Using a serrated knife, peel and thinly slice the remaining clementines. Roughly chop the nuts.
4 Fluff up the couscous with a fork, then mix in most of the nuts. Serve the couscous in bowls, topped with the clementines and raspberries. Eat with a spoonful of yogurt, an extra sprinkle of cinnamon and a squeeze of honey.

PER SERVING 333 kcals, fat 3g, saturates 1g, carbs 50g, sugars 16g, fibre 2g, protein 11g, salt 0.1g

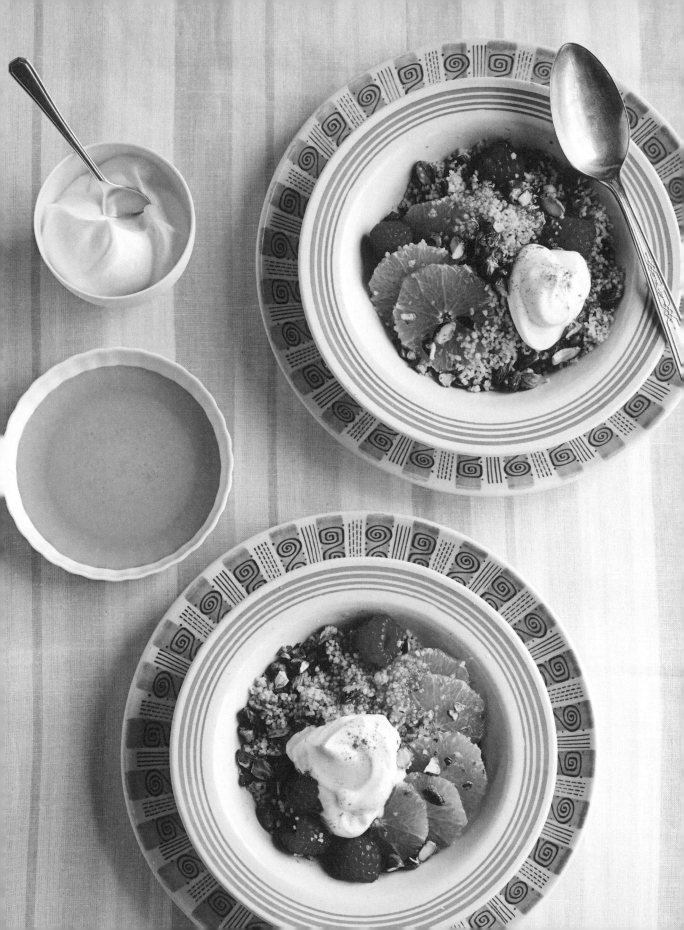

Berry Omelette Pancake

This delicious high-protein breakfast is a one-egg omelette cleverly disguised as a pancake. When berries are not in season try chopped banana with a sprinkle of cinnamon.

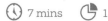 7 mins 1

- 1 large egg
- 1 tbsp skimmed milk
- 3 pinches of ground cinnamon
- ½ tsp rapeseed oil
- 100g/4oz cottage cheese
- 175g/6oz chopped strawberries, blueberries and raspberries

1 Beat the egg with the milk and cinnamon. Heat the oil in a 20cm non-stick frying pan and pour in the egg mixture, swirling to evenly cover the base. Cook for a few mins until set and golden underneath. There's no need to flip it over.

2 Place on a plate, spread over the cheese, then scatter with the berries. Roll up and serve.

PER SERVING 264 kcals, fat 12g, saturates 4g, carbs 18g, sugars 16g, fibre 4g, protein 21g, salt 1g

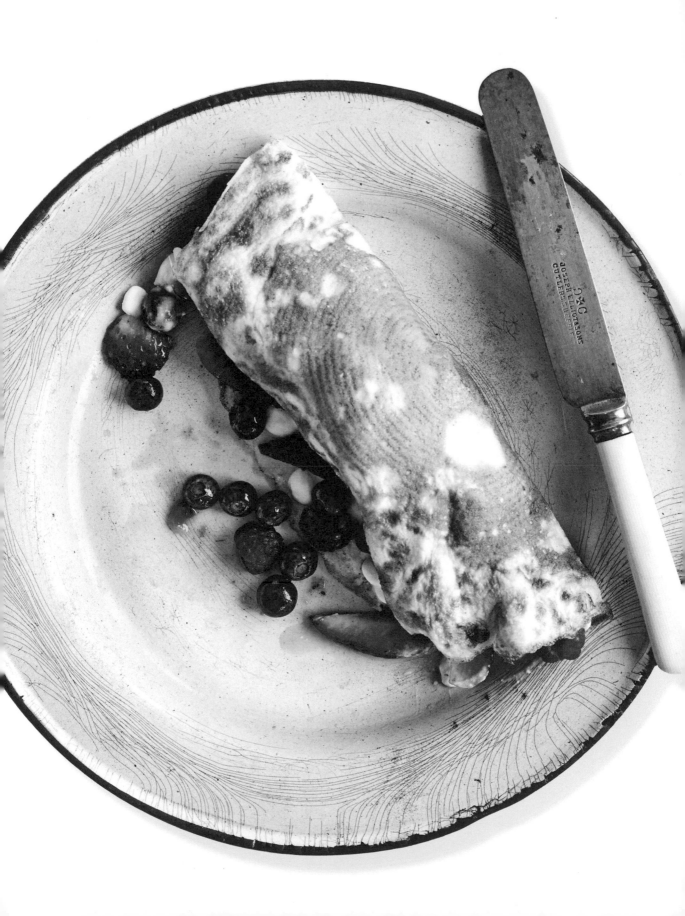

Omelette Pancakes with Tomato & Pepper Sauce

. . . .

Healthy, low-calorie and gluten-free these egg pancakes make a tasty brunch.

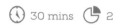 30 mins   2

- 4 large eggs
- handful fresh chopped basil

FOR THE TOMATO SAUCE

- 2 tsp rapeseed oil, plus a little extra for the pancakes
- 1 yellow pepper, quartered, deseeded and thinly sliced
- 2 garlic cloves, thinly sliced
- 1 tbsp white wine vinegar or cider vinegar
- 400g can chopped tomatoes
- wholemeal bread and salad leaves, to serve

1 First make the sauce. Heat the oil in a large frying pan and fry the pepper and garlic for 5 mins to soften them. Spoon in the vinegar and allow to sizzle away. Tip in the tomatoes then measure in a third of a can of water. Cover and leave to simmer for 10–15 mins until the peppers are tender and the sauce is nice and thick.

2 While it is cooking, make the pancakes. Beat an egg with 1 tsp water and seasoning then heat a small non-stick frying pan with a tiny amount of oil. Add the egg mixture and cook for about a min or two until set into a thin pancake. Lift onto a plate, cover with foil and carry on in the same way with the other eggs until you have 4 pancakes in total.

3 Roll up onto plates, spoon over the sauce and scatter with basil. Serve with bread or a handful of salad leaves on the side.

. . . .

PER SERVING 271 kcals, fat 17g, saturates 3g, carbs 11g, sugars 10g, fibre 4g, protein 19g, salt 0.6g

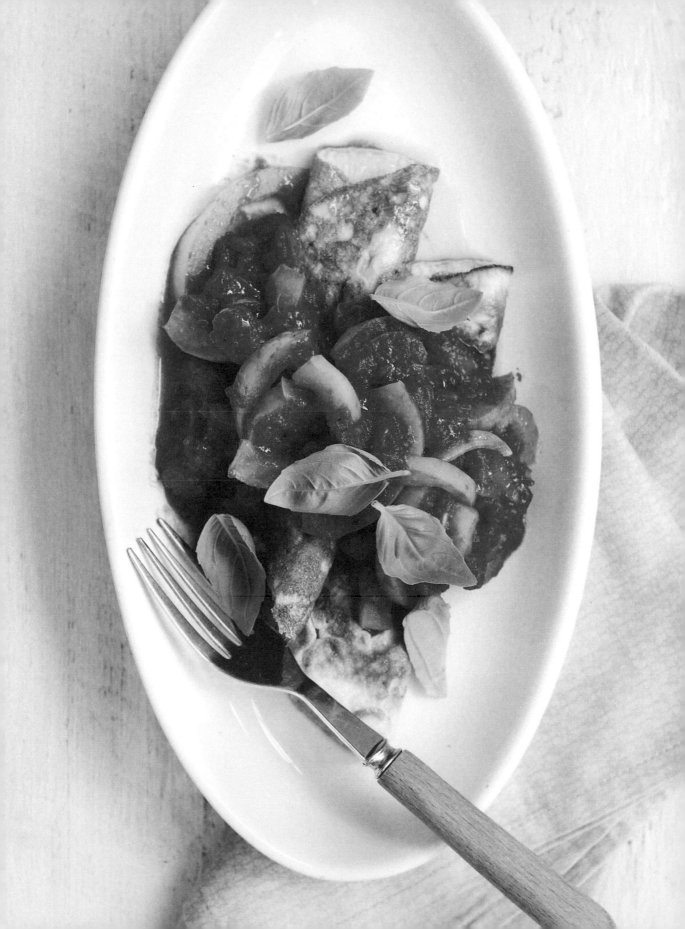

Veggie Breakfast Bakes

You can add a low-fat sausage or some rashers of turkey bacon to make this meaty, but still healthy, if you like.

🕐 45 mins   🥧 4

- 4 large field mushrooms
- 8 tomatoes, halved
- 1 garlic clove, thinly sliced
- 2 tsp olive or rapeseed oil
- 200g bag spinach leaves
- 4 eggs

1 Heat oven to 200C/180C fan/gas 6. Put the mushrooms and tomatoes into four ovenproof dishes. Divide the garlic among the dishes, drizzle over the oil and some seasoning, then bake for 10 mins.
2 Meanwhile, put the spinach into a large colander, then pour over a kettle of boiling water to wilt it. Squeeze out any excess water, then add the spinach to the dishes.
3 Make a little gap between the vegetables and crack an egg into each dish. Return to the oven and cook for a further 8–10 mins or until the egg is cooked to your liking.

PER SERVING 127 kcals, fat 8g, saturates 2g, carbs 5g, sugars 5g, fibre 3g, protein 9g, salt 0.4g

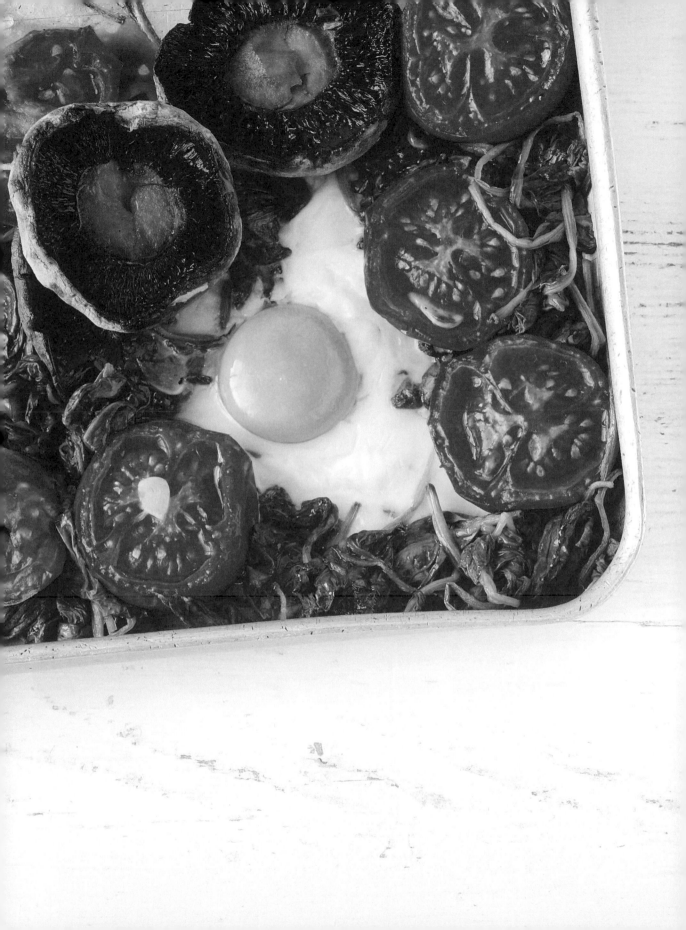

Egg & Tomato Baps

Don't butter the baps, simply squash on the hot tomatoes and sandwich with the herby omelette inside. Pour yourself a 150ml glass of orange juice to notch up 2 of your 5 a day.

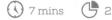 7 mins   2

- 2 tomatoes, halved
- 2 tsp olive or rapeseed oil
- 4 eggs
- couple of sprigs of parsley, chopped (optional)
- 1 garlic clove, finely chopped
- 2 wholewheat baps

1 Brush the cut sides of the tomatoes with a little of the oil then cook them cut side down in a small, non-stick frying pan. Meanwhile beat the eggs with seasoning and the chopped parsley. Turn the tomatoes over to briefly heat and cook the other side.
2 Wipe the pan, then add the remaining oil and cook the garlic for a few seconds, stirring all the time until softened. Pour in the egg mixture and cook, stirring occasionally over the heat. When two-thirds set, leave it to become an omelette then flip over to cook the other side for a few seconds more.
3 Halve the baps and squash on the tomatoes, quarter the omelette and serve, two pieces each, inside.

PER SERVING 323 kcals, fat 16g, saturates 4g, carbs 24g, sugars 4g, fibre 4g, protein 19g, salt 1g

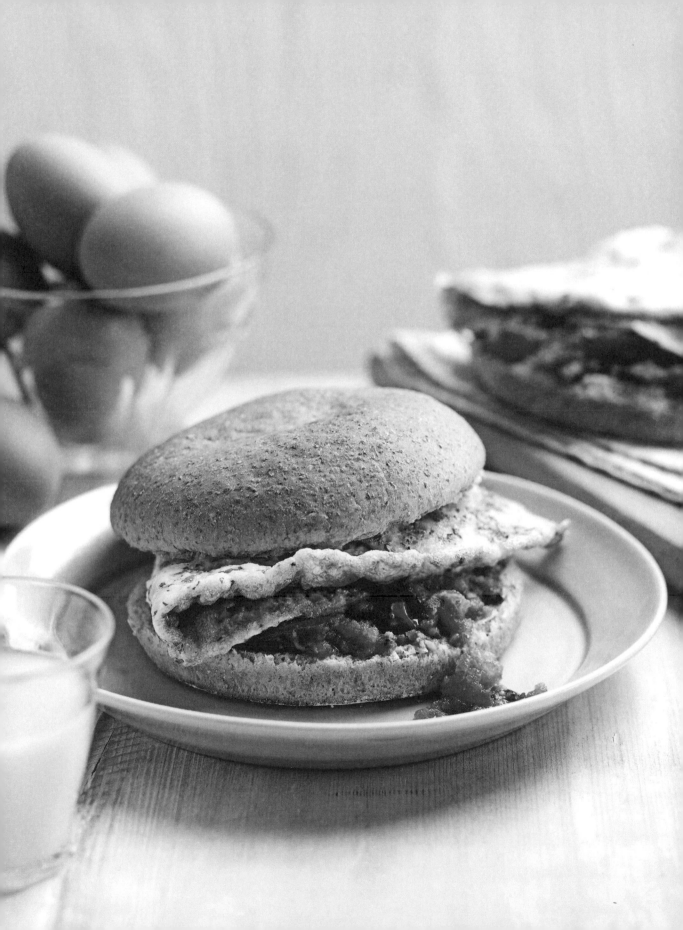

Dippy Eggs with Marmite Soldiers

Boiled eggs get a tasty makeover; remember though, the Marmite is quite salty, so use sparingly.

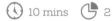 10 mins 2

- 2 eggs (to serve 1 egg per person)
- 4 slices wholemeal bread
- knob butter
- Marmite, for spreading
- mixed seeds, for dipping (optional)

1 Bring a pan of water to a simmer. Add the eggs, simmer for 2 mins if room temp, 3 mins if fridge-cold, then turn off the heat. Cover the pan and leave for 2 mins more.
2 Meanwhile, toast 4 slices wholemeal bread and spread thinly with butter, then Marmite. To serve, cut into soldiers and dip into the egg, then a few mixed seeds if you like.

PER SERVING 372 kcals, fat 21g, saturates 8g, carbs 31g, sugars 2g, fibre 4g, protein 17g, salt 1.09g

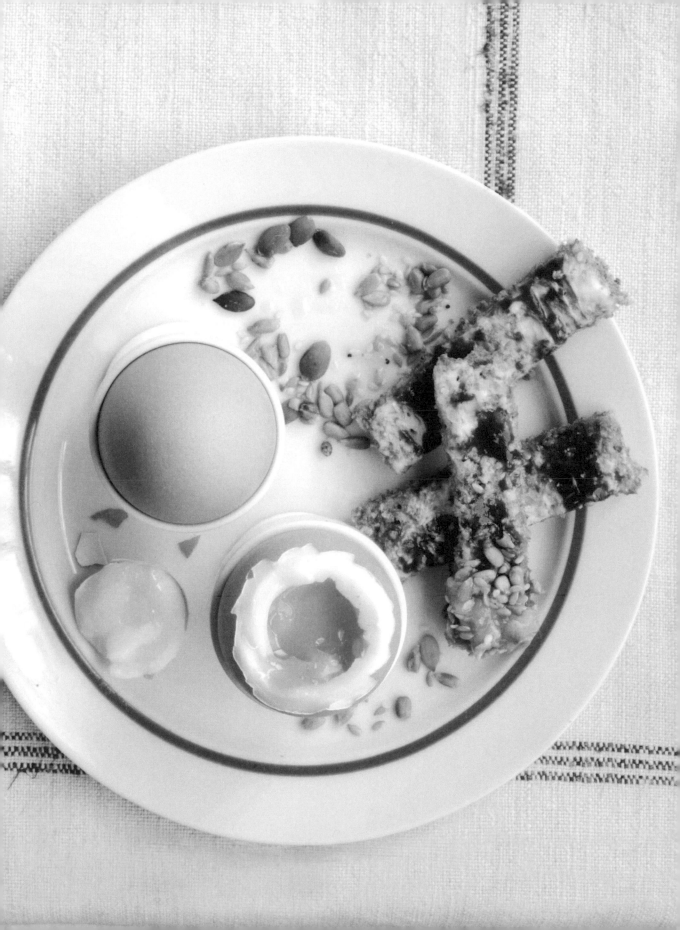

Kedgeree with Poached Eggs

We've used a budget-friendly fish pie mix – a combination of white and smoked fish chunks with salmon, rather than all smoked fish, to reduce the level of salt in this kedgeree.

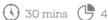 30 mins 4

- 300g/11oz long grain brown rice
- 2 tbsp olive oil
- 1 onion, finely chopped
- 2 garlic cloves, finely chopped
- 390g pack fish pie mix, defrosted if frozen
- 1 heaped tbsp mild or medium curry powder
- juice 1 lemon
- ¼ small pack parsley, chopped
- 4 eggs

1 Cook the rice following the pack instructions, then drain and set aside. Meanwhile, heat 1 tbsp of the oil in a non-stick frying pan and cook the onion and garlic for 5 mins. Toss the fish pieces with the curry powder and remaining oil. Add to the pan. Cook for another 5 mins, stirring carefully and turning the fish.

2 Add the rice to the pan and turn up the heat, then stir well (the fish will break up a little). Cook for 1-2 mins, then stir in the lemon and parsley. Turn the heat down as low as it will go, and put on a lid.

3 Bring a pan of water to the boil, turn down the heat and poach the eggs. Season the kedgeree and divide between plates, topping each with a poached egg.

PER SERVING 542 kcals, fat 17g, saturates 4g, carbs 63g, sugars 2g, fibre 3g, protein 31g, salt 1.07g

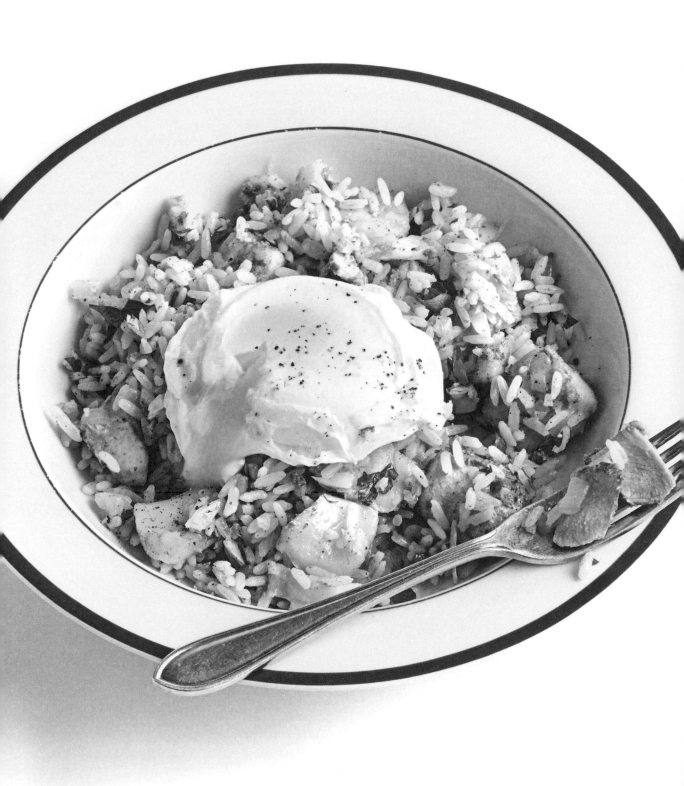

Broccoli & Poached Egg Toasts

This may sound like an unusual way to enjoy your eggs for brunch but broccoli is a super food and blood-sugar wonder.

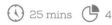 25 mins   4

- 225g/8oz purple sprouting broccoli
- 1 ciabatta loaf
- 1 garlic clove, halved
- 2 tbsp olive oil
- 1 tbsp Dijon mustard
- 6 shallots, halved lengthways
- 4 large eggs

1 Slice the broccoli and blanch in boiling water for 1 min. Drain and refresh in cold water. Dry on kitchen paper. Heat a griddle or frying pan.

2 Cut the ciabatta in half horizontally, then cut each slice in half. Rub with the garlic and brush with half the oil. Cook the ciabatta on the griddle for 1-2 minutes on each side until golden. Spread with mustard and keep warm.

3 Toss the shallots in the remaining olive oil and cook cut-side down on the griddle for 2 mins on each side. Keep warm.

4 Pile the broccoli on to the griddle and cook for 3-4 mins, turning frequently. Meanwhile, poach the eggs in gently simmering water until set to your liking. Pile the shallots and broccoli on the ciabatta. Top with the eggs and season.

PER SERVING 350 kcals, fat 14g, saturates 3g, carbs 36g, sugars 4g, fibre 4g, protein 17g, salt 1.6g

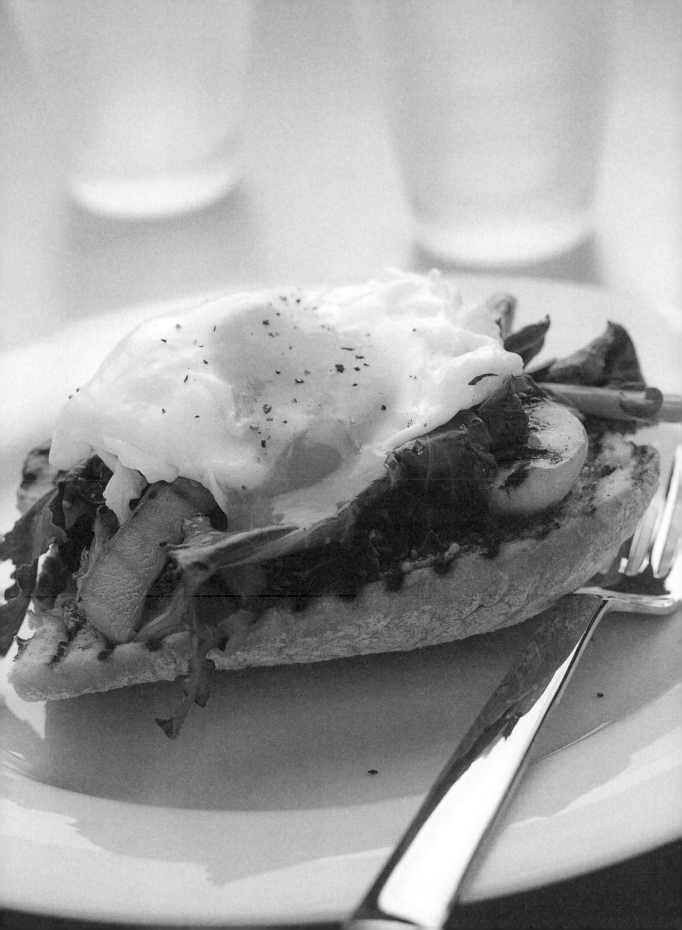

Smoky Beans on Toast

Forget shop-bought cans of baked beans, this homemade version is tastier and healthier, and includes an impressive 4 of your 5 a day.

🕐 35 mins   🥧 2 generously

- 1 tbsp olive or rapeseed oil
- 1 small onion, sliced
- 1 small red pepper, deseeded and thinly sliced
- 1 garlic clove, halved
- 400g can chopped tomatoes
- 1 tsp smoked paprika
- 2 tsp red or white wine vinegar
- 400g can butter beans
- ¼ tsp sugar (optional)
- 2 slices seed bread
- few parsley sprigs, finely chopped (optional)

1 Heat the oil in a pan, add the onion and pepper and fry gently until soft, about 10-15 mins. Crush half the garlic and add this to the pan, along with the tomatoes, paprika, vinegar, beans and their juice, sugar, if using, and some seasoning. Bring to a simmer and cook for 10-15 mins or until slightly reduced and thickened.

2 Toast the bread, rub with the remaining garlic and drizzle with a little oil. Spoon the beans over the toast and scatter over the parsley, if using.

PER SERVING 460 kcals, fat 19g, saturates 3g, carbs 49g, sugars 17g, fibre 14g, protein 15g, salt 1.1g

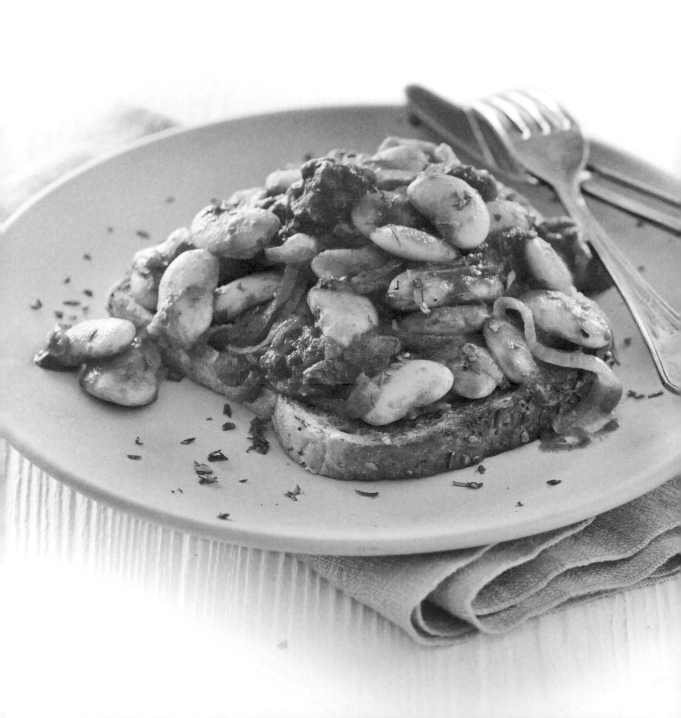

Creamy Mustard Mushrooms on Toast served with Orange Juice

Adding a 150ml glass of fruit juice means this breakfast contributes 2 of your 5 a day. However, even unsweetened juice is rich in natural sugars so don't be tempted to exceed it.

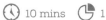 10 mins 1

- 1 slice wholemeal bread
- 1½ tbsp light cream cheese
- 1 tsp rapeseed oil
- 3 handfuls of sliced, small flat mushrooms
- 2 tbsp skimmed milk
- ¼ tsp wholegrain mustard
- 1 tbsp snipped chives
- 150ml/¼ pint orange juice, freshly squeezed or from a carton

1 Toast the bread then spread with a little of the cheese instead of using butter.
2 Meanwhile, heat the oil in a non-stick pan, add the mushrooms and cook, stirring frequently until they have softened.
3 Spoon in the the milk, remaining cheese and the mustard and stir well until coated. Tip onto the toast and top with the chives. Serve with a glass of orange juice.

PER SERVING 231 kcals, fat 7g, saturates 2g, carbs 28g, sugars 16g, fibre 4g, protein 13g, salt 0.1g

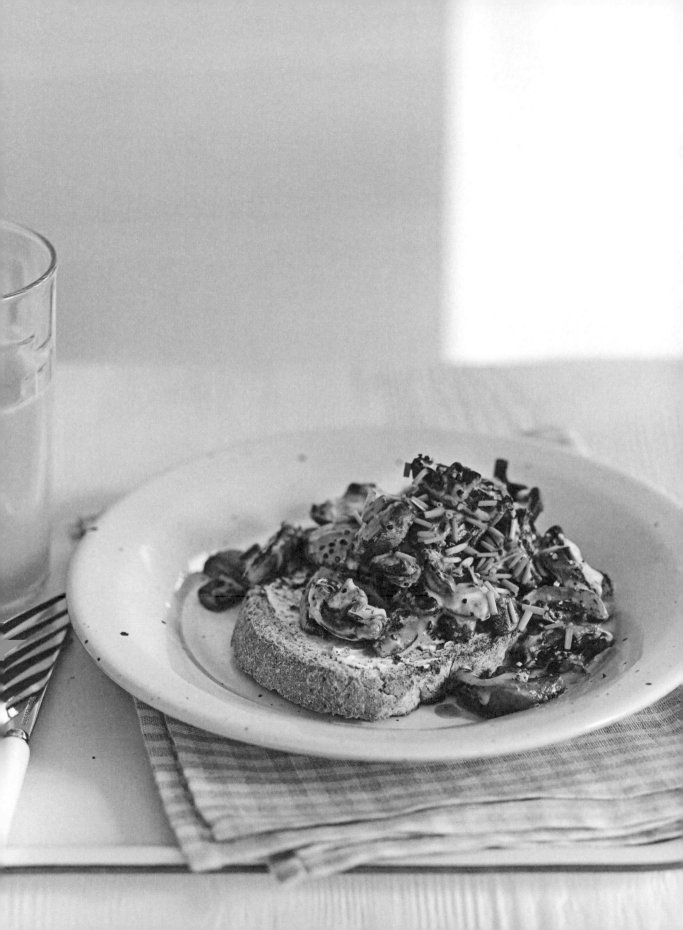

Smoky Rashers & Tomatoes on Toast

Turkey rashers are a great low-fat alternative for bacon while mashed avocado provides a nutritious alternative to butter.

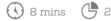 8 mins 2

- rapeseed oil, for frying
- 4 smoked turkey rashers
- 3 tomatoes, halved
- 2 slices whole wheat bread
- 1 tsp English mustard
- 1 small ripe avocado
- 2 handfuls rocket

1 Heat a non-stick pan or griddle and spray or rub with a little oil to lightly grease it. Cook the turkey rashers and tomatoes for a couple of minutes on each side.

2 Meanwhile, toast the bread, spread with mustard and squash half an avocado on top. Pile on the turkey rashers and tomatoes with the rocket and serve while still hot.

PER SERVING 269 kcals, fat 13g, saturates 3g, carbs 19g, sugars 6g, fibre 6g, protein 19g, salt 1.7g

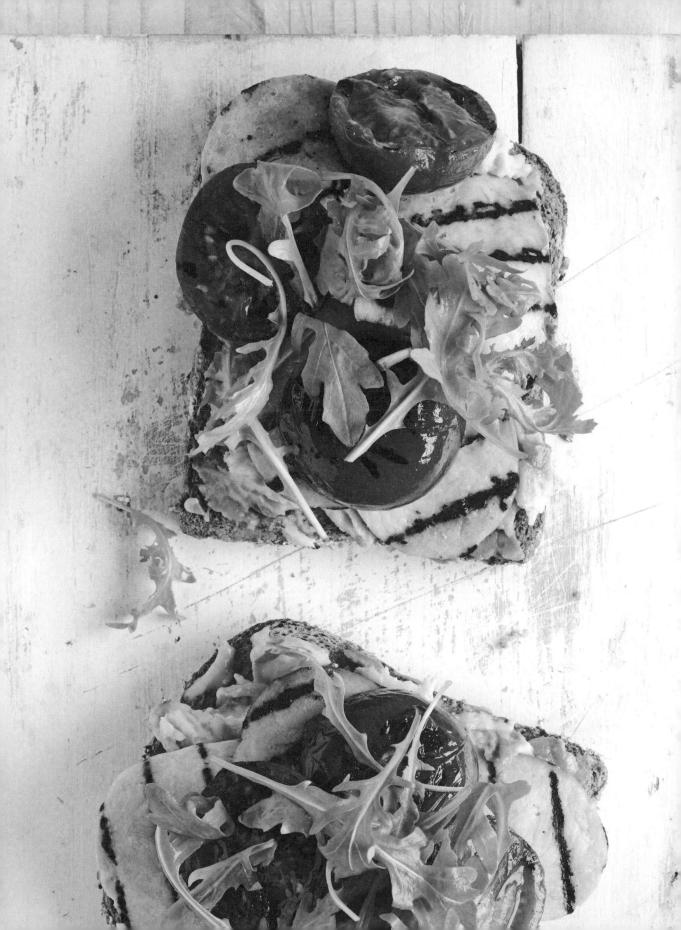

Almond Butter

Blitz up your own homemade nut butter for spreading on toast for a speedy breakfast, filling pancakes or adding to sauces and smoothies.

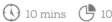 10 mins  10

- 250g/9oz blanched almonds
- 2 tbsp mild oil, such as olive, coconut or almond oil

1 Put the almonds in a food processor and blitz on high speed until finely chopped and the nuts have come together to form a thick ball. With the processor still running, add the oil, a little at a time, until the mixture is a smooth, glossy paste – about 7 mins.

2 Spoon into a clean jar, and keep tightly closed and refrigerated when not in use. Will keep in the fridge for up to 3 weeks.

PER SERVING 158 kcals, fat 15g, saturates 1g, carbs 2g, sugars 1g, fibre 2g, protein 5g, salt none

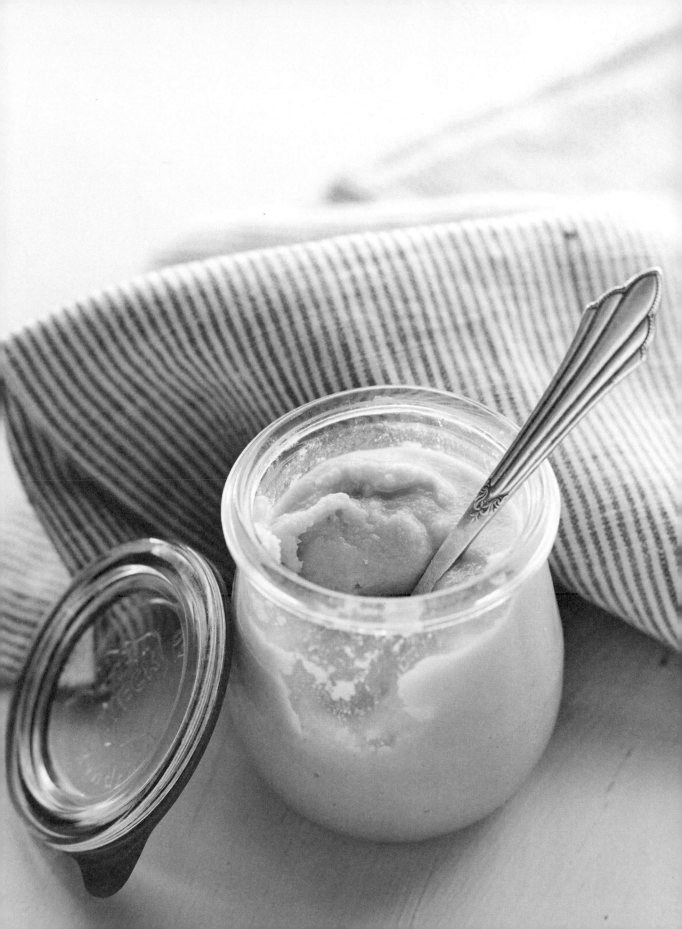

Rye Bread with Almond Butter & Pink Grapefruit

A balanced breakfast of rye toast, with homemade nut butter and juicy fruit.

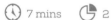 7 mins 2

- 2 slices rye bread (see recipe page 268)
- 1 pink grapefruit
- 4 tbsp almond butter, bought or homemade (see page 42)

1 Toast your rye bread, if you like. Segment the grapefruit and spoon the fruit, along with any juice, into a small bowl.

2 Spread the almond butter onto the rye bread, and top with the grapefruit, drizzling any juice over the top.

PER SERVING 333 kcals, fat 18g, saturates 2g, carbs 30g, sugars 7g, fibre 8g, protein 10g, salt 0.8g

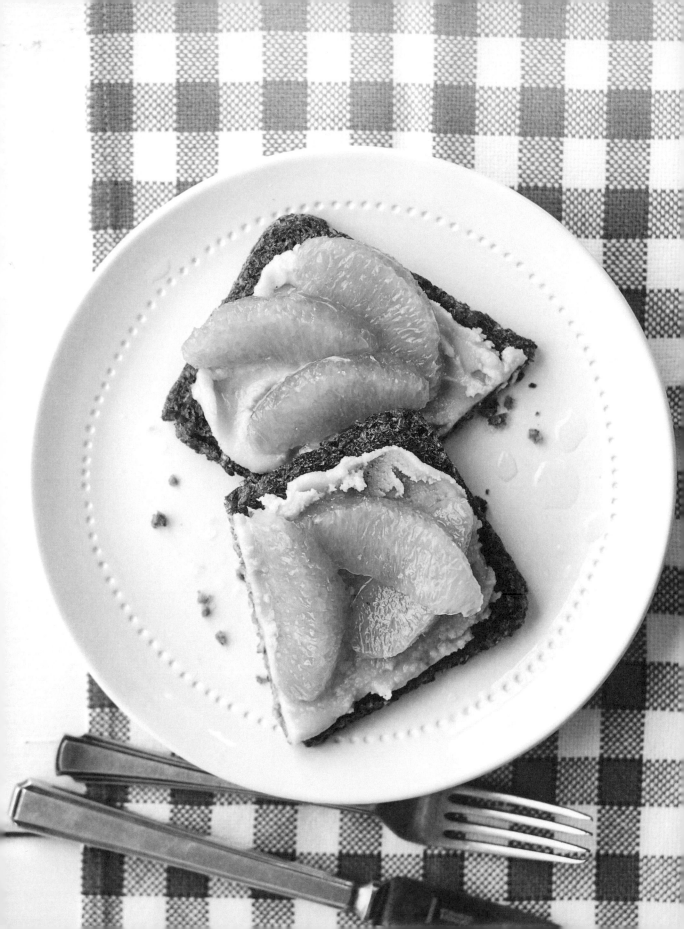

Breakfast Muffins

Make muffins healthier with mashed banana and apple sauce for natural sweetness, plus blueberries and seeds for an extra nutritious hit. You can even use homemade stewed apple.

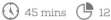 45 mins   12

- 2 large eggs
- 150ml pot natural low-fat yogurt
- 50ml/2floz rapeseed oil
- 100g/4oz apple sauce (find with baby food)
- 1 ripe banana, mashed
- 4 tbsp clear honey
- 1 tsp vanilla extract
- 200g/7oz plain wholemeal flour
- 50g/2oz rolled oats, plus extra for sprinkling
- 1½ tsp baking powder
- 1½ tsp bicarbonate of soda
- 1½ tsp ground cinnamon
- 100g/4oz fresh or frozen blueberries
- 2 tbsp mixed seeds (we used pumpkin, sunflower and linseed)

1 Heat oven to 180C/160C fan/gas 4. Line a 12-hole muffin tin with 12 large muffin cases or squares of baking parchment. In a jug, mix the eggs, yogurt, oil, apple sauce, banana, honey and vanilla. Tip the remaining ingredients, except the seeds, into a large bowl, add a pinch of salt and mix to combine.

2 Pour the wet ingredients into the dry and mix briefly until you have smooth batter – don't over mix as this will make the muffins heavy. Divide the batter between the cases. Sprinkle the muffins with the extra oats and the seeds. Bake for 25-30 mins until golden and well risen, and a skewer inserted into the centre of a muffin comes out clean. Remove from the oven, transfer to a wire rack and leave to cool. Can be stored in a sealed container for up to 3 days.

PER MUFFIN 179 kcals, fat 7g, saturates 1g, carbs 23g, sugars 10g, fibre 3g, protein 5g, salt 0.06g

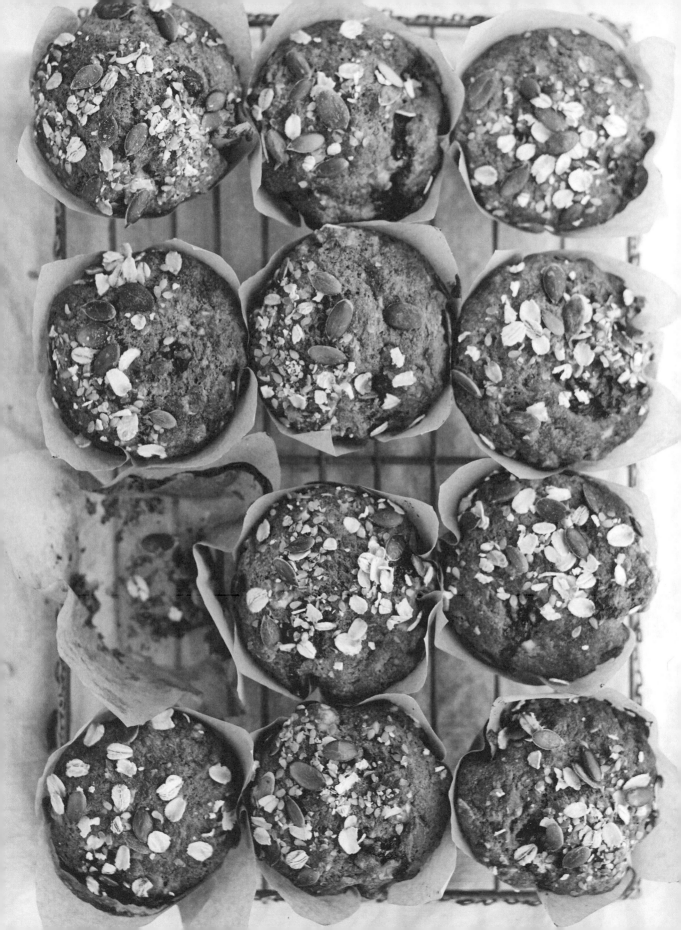

Fig & Nut Seed Bread

Keep this in the fridge, or portion the slices for the freezer for a great breakfast when you are short of time. Top with ricotta or low-fat soft cheese and fresh fruit instead of butter.

🕐 1½ hours   ◔ cuts into 16

- 400ml/14fl oz hot strong black tea
- 100g/4oz dried figs, hard stalks removed, thinly sliced
- 140g/5oz sultanas
- 50g/2oz oats
- 200g/7oz self-raising whole wheat flour
- 1 tsp baking powder
- 100g/4oz mixed nuts (almonds, walnuts, Brazils, hazelnuts), plus 50g/2oz for the top
- 1 tbsp each golden linseeds and sesame, plus 2 tsp sesame to sprinkle
- 25g/1oz pumpkin seeds
- 1 large egg
- 25g/1oz ricotta for spreading and 1 thickly sliced orange or green apple per serving

1 Heat oven to 170C/150C fan/gas 3½. Pour the tea into a large bowl and stir in the figs, sultanas and oats. Set aside to soak while you get on with the rest of the loaf.

2 Line the base and sides of a 900g/1lb loaf tin with baking parchment. Mix the flour, baking powder, 100g nuts and the seeds. Beat the egg into the cooled fruit mixture then stir the dried ingredients in to the wet. Pile into the tin then level the top and scatter with the remaining nuts and sesame seeds.

3 Bake for 1 hour then cover the top with foil and bake for 15 mins more until a skewer inserted into the centre of the loaf comes out clean. Remove from the tin to cool, but leave the paper on until cold. Serve sliced spread with ricotta rather than butter, which is lower in fat and higher in protein and fruit. It will keep in the fridge for a month.

PER SERVING 249 kcals, fat 10g, saturates 3g, carbs 30g, sugars 20g, fibre 6g, protein 10g, salt 0.3g

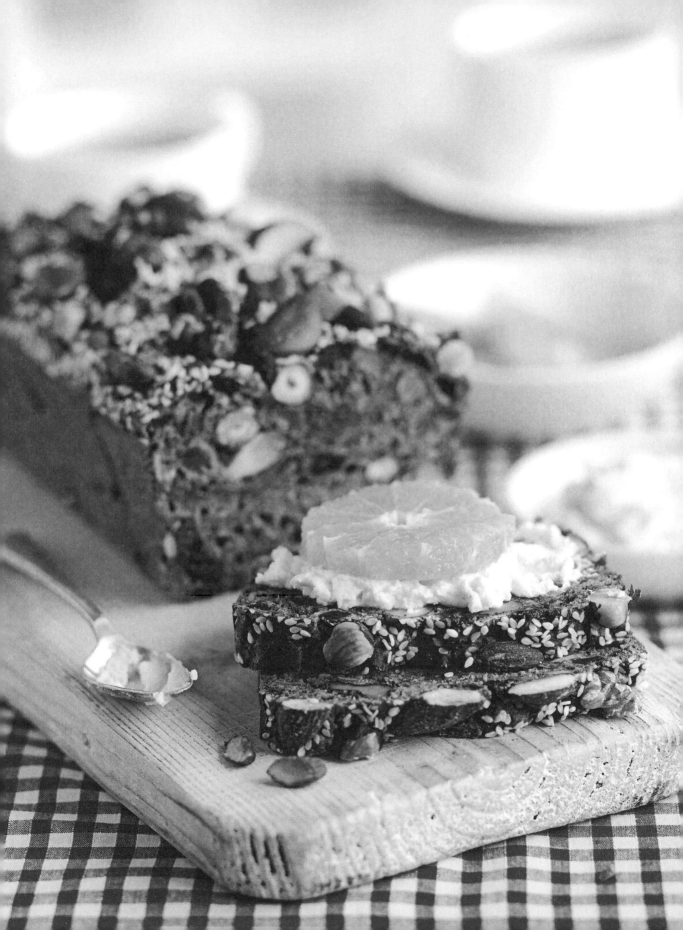

Strawberry & Banana Almond Smoothie

Ground almonds makes this breakfast in a glass surprisingly filling as well as balancing the natural sugars in the fruit. This will start your day off with 2 of your 5 a day.

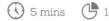 5 mins 1

- 1 small banana
- 7 strawberries, fresh or frozen, hulled
- 3 tbsp 0%-fat bio yogurt
- 3 tbsp skimmed milk
- 2 tbsp ground almonds

1 Slice the banana into a jug if using a hand-held blender or the bowl of a food processor. Add the berries, yogurt, milk and ground almonds then blitz until completely smooth. Pour into a glass and enjoy!

PER SMOOTHIE 373 kcals, fat 17.4g, saturates 1.6g, carbs 35.8g, sugars 32.9g, fibre 2.4g, protein 17.1g, salt 0.3g

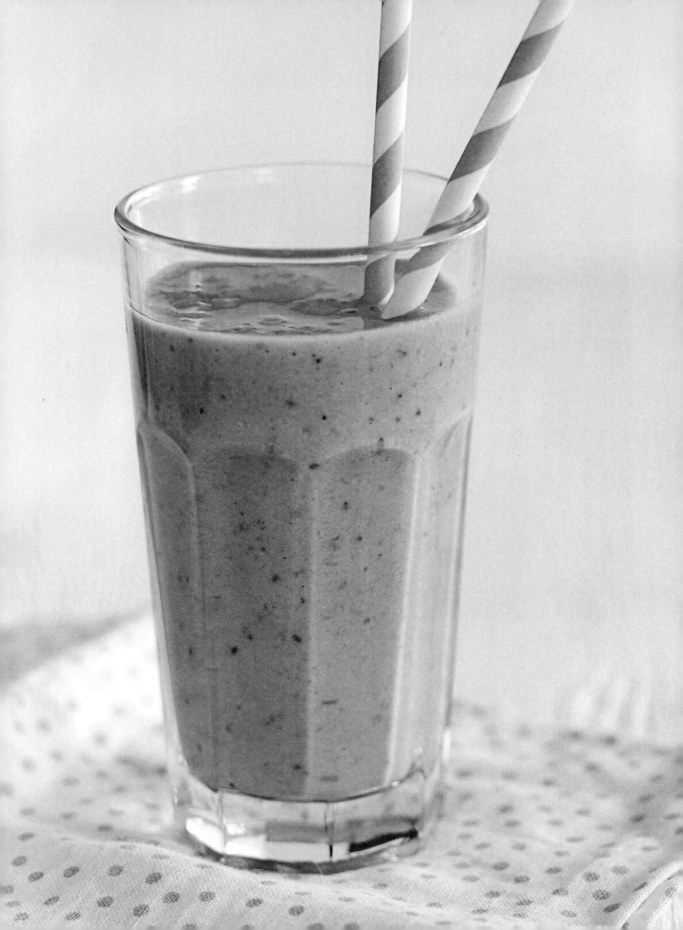

Minty Pineapple Smoothie

There's more to smoothies than just fruit – this dairy-free green blend contains spinach, oats, linseeds and cashew nuts, too. Use canned pineapple in fruit juice, if you like instead of fresh.

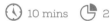 10 mins 2

- 200g/7oz pineapple, peeled, cored and cut into chunks
- a few mint leaves
- 50g/2oz baby spinach leaves
- 25g/1oz oats
- 2 tbsp linseeds
- handful unsalted, cashew nuts
- fresh lime juice, to taste

1 Put all the ingredients in a blender with 200ml water and process until smooth. If it's too thick, add more water (up to 400ml) until you get the right mix.

PER SERVING 177 kcals, fat 8g, saturates 1g, carbs 19g, sugars 11g, fibre 4g, protein 6g, salt 0.1g

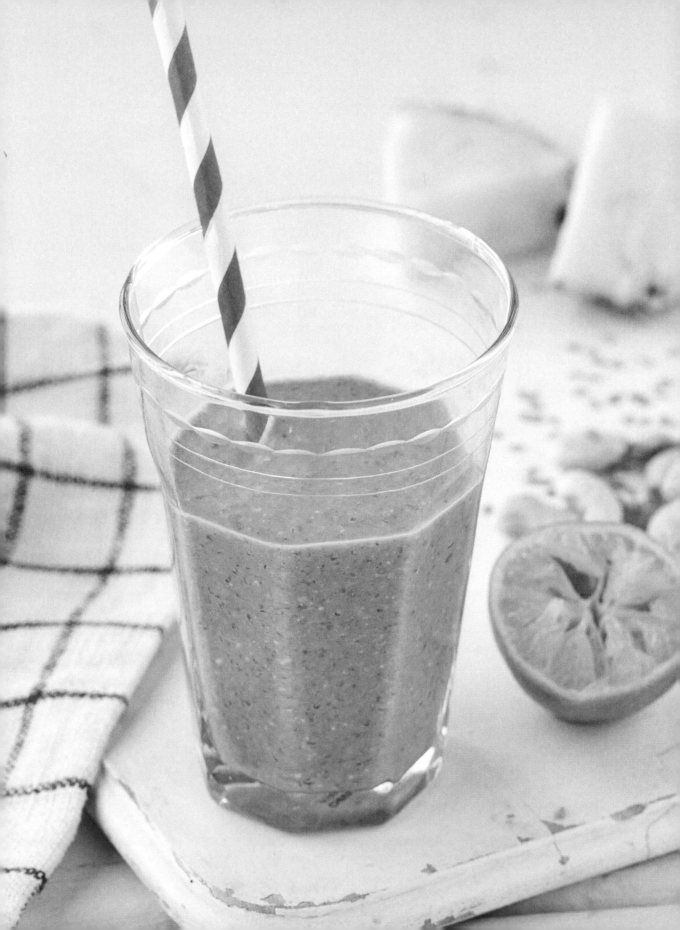

Pick Me Up Smoothie

This breakfast in a glass is also ideal to serve in the afternoon, when you can feel yourself lagging but it's nowhere near supper time.

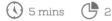 5 mins   2

- 500ml/18fl oz unsweetened almond milk or semi-skimmed milk
- 2 tbsp almond butter (see recipe page 42)
- 6 pitted prunes
- 1 tsp ground cinnamon
- 1 small ripe banana

1 In a blender, whizz the milk with the almond butter, prunes, cinnamon and banana. Chill until ready to drink, or pack for a snack on the go. They will keep in the fridge for 2 days.

PER SERVING 250 kcals, fat 11g, saturates 1g, carbs 29g, sugars 22g, fibre 5g, protein 5g, salt 0.3g

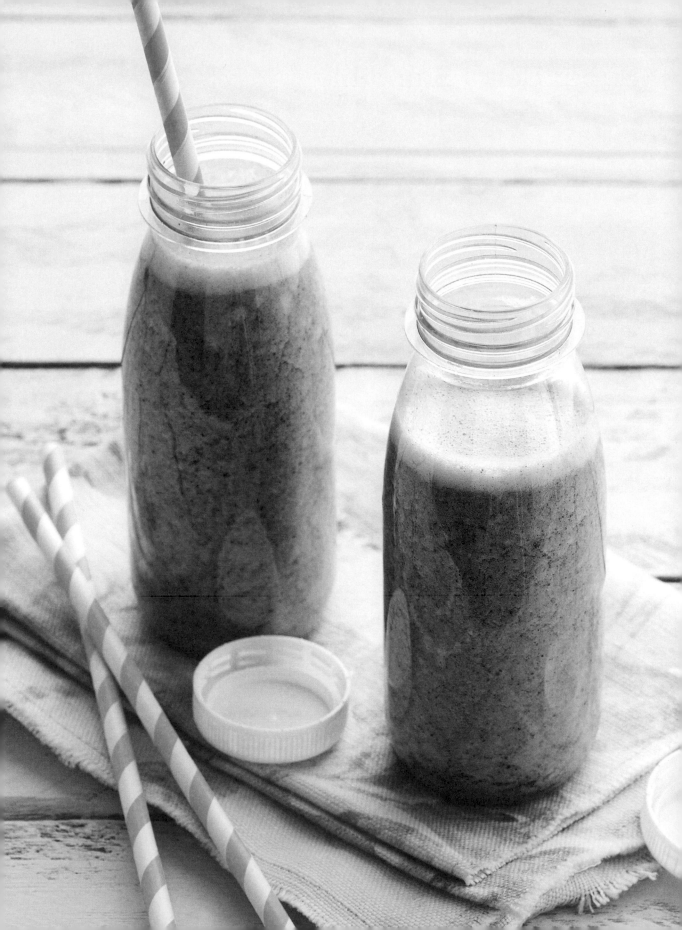

Super Berry Smoothie

Use frozen berries for a thrifty way of creating a healthy smoothie that is nice and cold to drink, too.

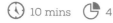 10 mins 4

- 450g/1lb frozen berries
- 450g pot fat-free strawberry yogurt
- 100ml/3½fl oz milk
- 25g/1oz porridge oats
- 2 tsp honey (optional)

1 Whizz the berries, yogurt and milk together in a food processor or with a stick blender until smooth. Stir through the porridge oats, then pour into 4 glasses and serve with a drizzle of honey, if you like.

PER SERVING 117 kcals, fat 1g, saturates 1g, carbs 18g, sugars 14g, fibre 4g, protein 8g, salt 0.2g

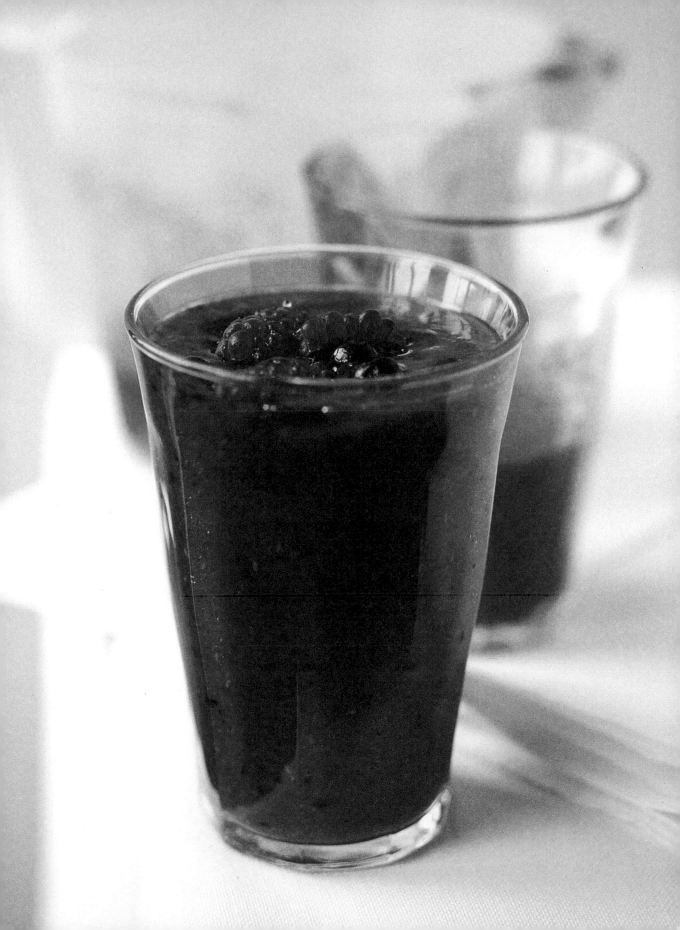

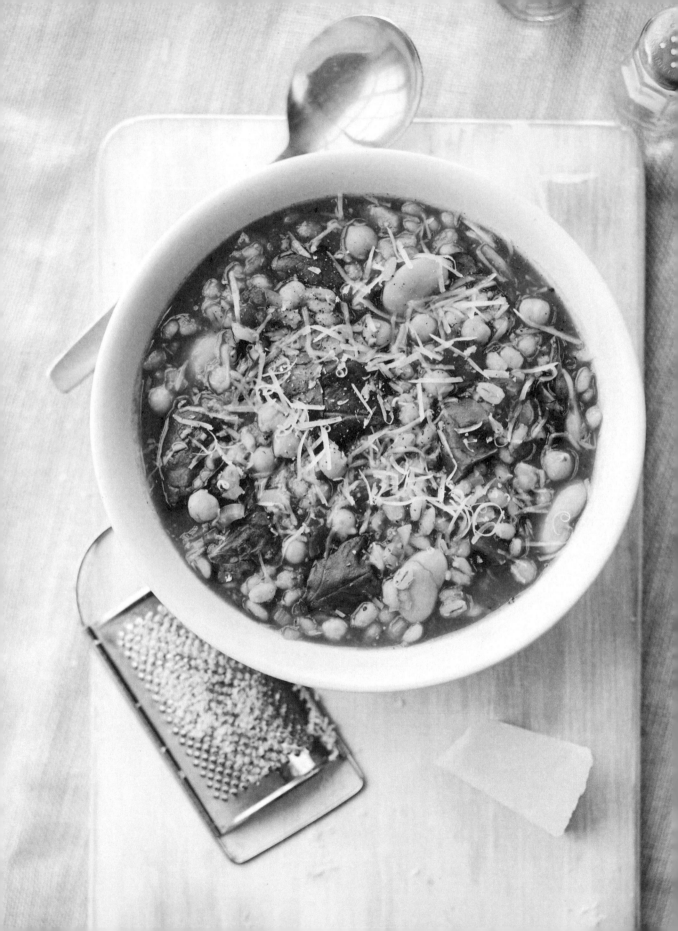

Chapter 2:

SUBSTANTIAL SOUPS & SNACKS

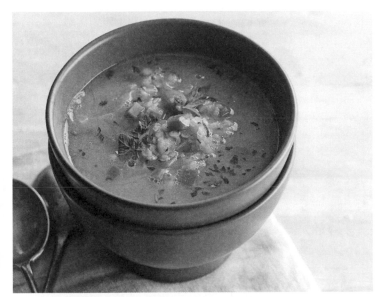

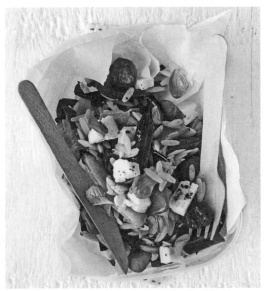

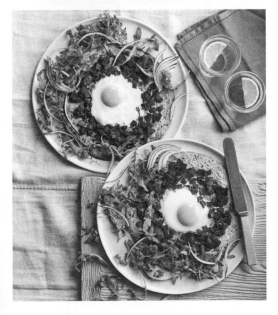

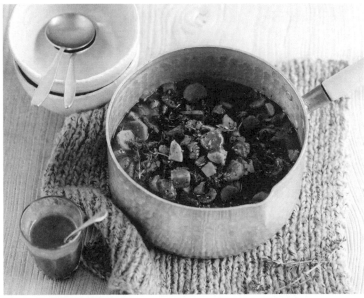

Bone Broth

Don't throw away a chicken carcass, it makes a really nourishing, tasty soup full of amino acids, gelatin (good for the joints) and minerals. Brown rice makes it more substantial.

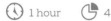 1 hour 4

- 1 meaty leftover chicken carcass, skin removed
- 1 large onion, halved and sliced
- grated zest and juice of 1 lemon
- 2 bay leaves, fresh or dried
- 1-2 red chillies, halved deseeded and sliced
- 1 tsp ground coriander
- ½ tsp ground cumin
- small pack fresh coriander, stems and leaves chopped but kept apart
- 1 large garlic clove, finely grated
- 250g pouch brown basmati rice

1 Break the chicken carcass into a large pan then add the onion, 1½ litres water, the lemon juice and bay leaves. Cover the pan and simmer for 40 mins. Remove from the heat and allow it to cool slightly.

2 Place a colander over a bowl then scoop out all of the bones into the colander and pick through them, stripping off the chicken and returning it to the pan with any onion as you work your way down the pile of bones.

3 Return any broth from the bowl to the pan with the chillies, ground coriander, cumin, fresh coriander stems, lemon zest and garlic and cook for a few mins until just bubbling – don't boil hard as you will spoil the delicate flavours. Season only if you need to.

4 Meanwhile heat the rice according to the pack and toss with the chopped coriander leaves. Ladle the broth into bowls, top with the rice and serve.

PER SERVING 150 kcals, fat 3g, saturates 1g, carbs 24g, sugars 5g, fibre 2g, protein 6g, salt 0.9g

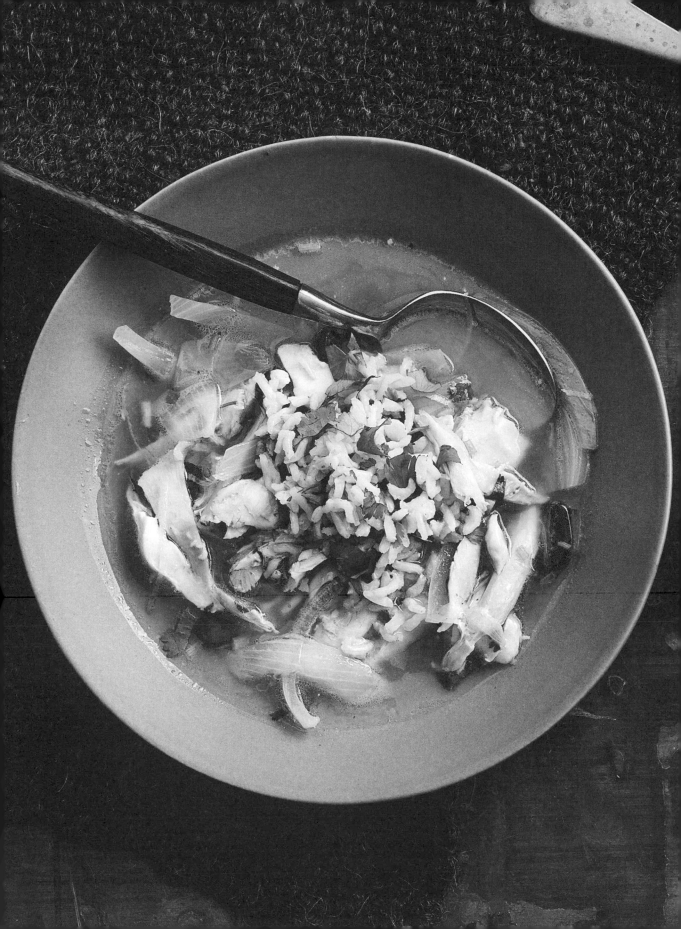

Herby Chicken & Butter Bean Soup

This good for you soup freezes well for up to 6 weeks so you can pack some away for another meal. If you don't have fresh herbs use 1 tsp each dried, although fresh give the best flavour.

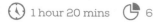 1 hour 20 mins 6

- 1 leftover chicken carcass plus up to 225g/8oz meat, roughly chopped
- 2 tbsp rapeseed oil
- 2 onions, chopped
- 6 carrots, chopped
- 3-4 sprigs each rosemary, sage and thyme, leaves picked and chopped
- 2 tsp each ground cumin and coriander
- 1 tsp turmeric
- 1 tbsp plain flour
- 400g can butter beans, rinsed and drained

1 Put the chicken carcass, in a large pan and cover with 2 litres of water. Bring to the boil, then cover with a lid and gently simmer for 20 mins.

2 Meanwhile, heat the oil in another large pan, add the onions and cook for 10 mins until starting to caramelise. Add the carrots, herbs, spices and flour, and stir for 1-2 mins to toast the spices. Strain the cooking liquid from the carcass into the pan with the vegetables. Stir well, cover and simmer for 30 mins.

3 Add the chicken meat to the soup along with the butter beans, season and heat through for 1-2 mins. Serve as it is or puree half with a hand-held blender so it's creamy but still has chunks of chicken, carrot and butter beans.

PER SERVING 363 kcals, fat 19g, saturates 4g, carbs 19g, sugars 11g, fibre 7g, protein 32g, salt 0.8g

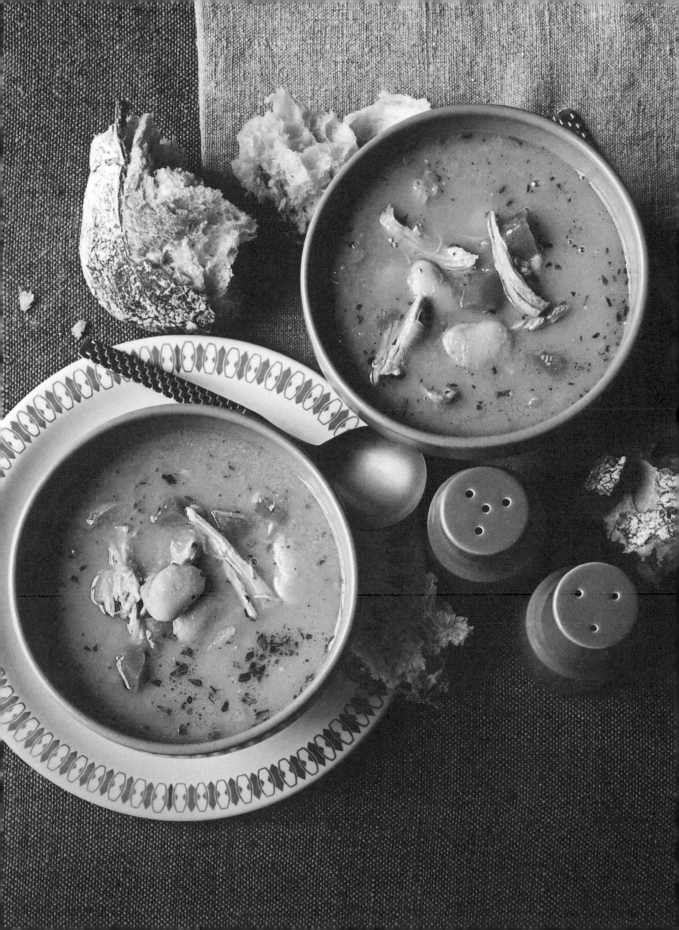

Spiced Black Bean & Chicken Soup with Kale

Wholesome and hearty, this South American-style recipe providing 2 of your 5 a day has plenty of pep from store cupboard spices and rich-tasting kale.

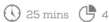 25 mins 4

- 2 tbsp rapeseed oil
- 2 fat garlic cloves, crushed
- small bunch coriander, stalks finely chopped, leaves picked
- zest 1 lime, then cut into wedges
- 2 tsp ground cumin
- 1 tsp chilli flakes
- 400g can chopped tomatoes
- 400g can black beans, rinsed and drained
- 600ml/1 pint chicken stock
- 175g/6oz shredded kale
- 250g/9oz leftover chicken
- 50g/2oz feta, crumbled (optional)

1 Heat the oil in a large saucepan, add the garlic, coriander stalks and lime zest, then fry for 2 mins until fragrant. Stir in the cumin and chilli flakes, fry for 1 min more, then tip in the tomatoes, beans and stock. Bring to the boil, then crush the beans against the bottom of the pan a few times using a potato masher. This will thicken the soup a little.

2 Stir the kale into the soup, simmer for 5 mins or until tender, then tear in the chicken and let it heat through. Season with the juice from half the lime, then serve in shallow bowls, scattered with the feta and a few coriander leaves. Serve the remaining lime in wedges for the table. The longer you leave the chicken in the pan, the thicker the soup will become, so add a splash more stock if you can't serve the soup straight away.

PER SERVING 293 kcals, fat 11g, saturates 2g, carbs 15g, sugars 3g, fibre 6g, protein 29g, salt 1.0g

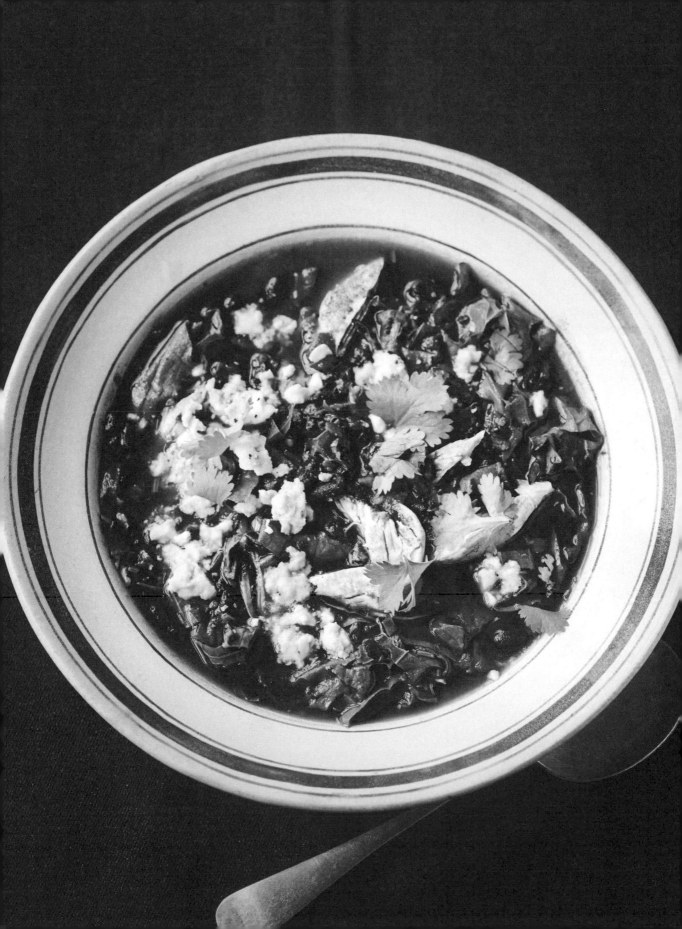

Jamaican Red Bean Soup

One steak serves two in this soup. Hot pepper sauce adds the authentic flavour; if you like a little heat use the rest of the bottle to splash onto cheese on toast or grilled meats and fish.

 30 mins 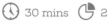 2

- 1 tsp rapeseed oil
- 175g/6oz lean rump steak, diced
- 1 small sweet potato, diced
- 2 small carrots, sliced
- 1 green pepper, deseeded and diced
- 1 celery stick, sliced
- 4 spring onions, thinly sliced
- 4 sprigs fresh thyme, leaves picked or ½ tsp dried
- 400g red kidney beans in water, no need to drain
- 600ml/1 pint beef stock
- hot pepper sauce, to taste

1 Heat the oil in a large non-stick pan and stir-fry the beef for 1 min until it just changes colour then take from the pan with a slotted spoon and set aside. Tip in all of the vegetables, add the thyme and fry for 5 mins until starting to soften.

2 Add in the beans and their juices with the stock and hot pepper sauce then cover and cook for 20 mins. Stir in the beef, cook for a few mins to heat through then serve in bowls.

PER SERVING 415 kcals, fat 8g, saturates 2g, carbs 39g, sugars 15g, fibre 18g, protein 38g, salt 1.7g

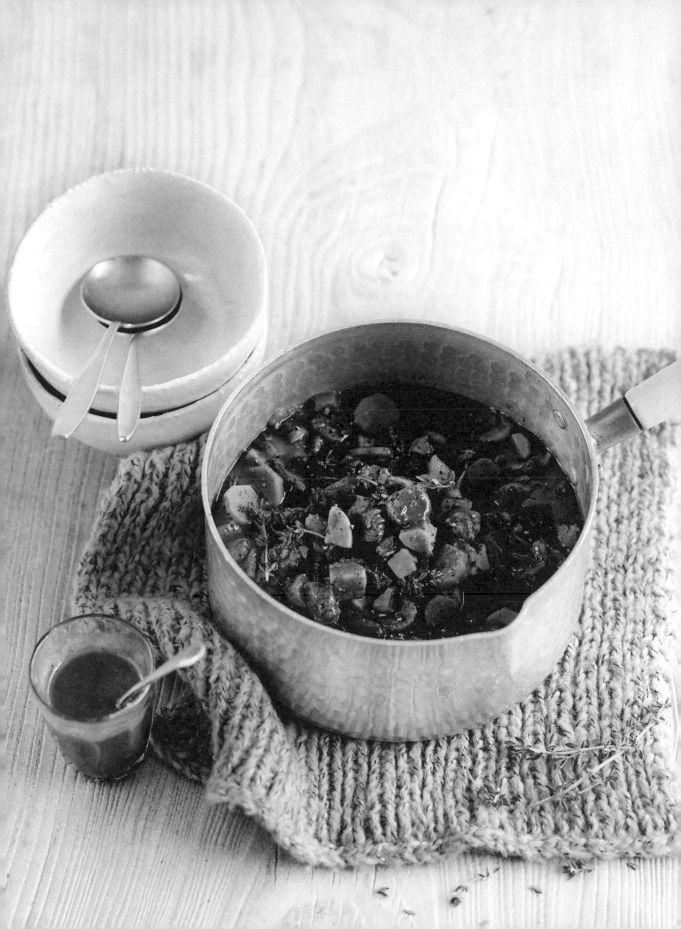

Bean & Barley Soup

Three of your 5 a day are packed into this chunky tomato-based soup. Barley, like oats, is good for the heart as it helps reduce cholesterol and blood pressure.

🕐 1 hr 5 mins   🥧 4

- 2 tbsp rapeseed oil
- 1 large onion, finely chopped
- 1 fennel bulb, quartered, cored and sliced or 3 celery sticks, sliced
- 5 garlic cloves, crushed
- 400g can chickpeas, rinsed drained
- 2 x 400g cans chopped tomatoes
- ½ tsp dried thyme or rosemary
- 600ml/1 pint vegetable stock
- 250g/9oz pearl barley
- 215g can butter beans, rinsed and drained
- 100g pack baby spinach leaves
- grated Parmesan, to serve

1 Heat the oil in a saucepan over a medium heat, add the onion, fennel or celery, herbs and garlic, and cook until softened and just beginning to brown, about 10-12 mins.

2 Mash half the chickpeas and add to the pan with the tomatoes, stock and barley. Top up with a can of water and bring to the boil, then reduce the heat and simmer, covered, for 45 mins or until the barley is tender. Add another can of water if the liquid has significantly reduced.

3 Add the remaining chickpeas and the butter beans to the soup. After a few mins, stir in the spinach and cook until wilted, about 1 min. Season and serve scattered with Parmesan.

PER SERVING 488 kcals, fat 9g, saturates 1g, carbs 78g, sugars 11g, fibre 12g, protein 16g, salt 1.4g

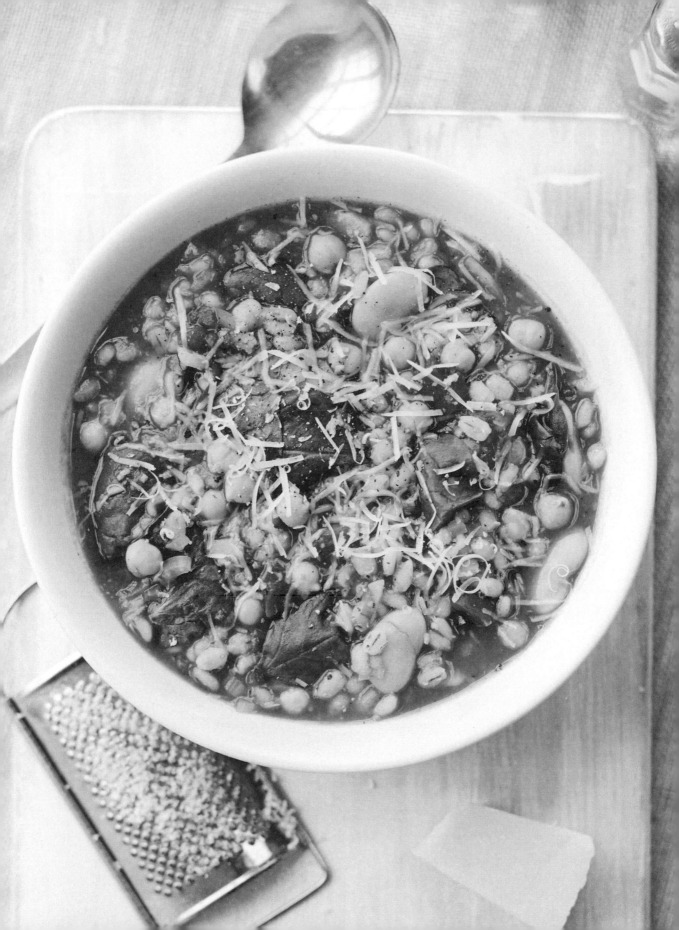

Red Lentil & Carrot Soup

This soup can be thrown together from ingredients most of us have in store and it's a good base for any veg left in the fridge.

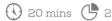 20 mins 2

- 2 tsp rapeseed oil
- 1 onion, sliced
- 3 garlic cloves, sliced
- 2 carrots, scrubbed and diced
- 85g/3oz red lentils
- 1 vegetable stock cube, crumbled
- 2 tbsp chopped parsley, plus a few extra leaves (optional)

1 Heat the oil in a medium pan, add the onion and fry for 2 mins. Add the garlic and carrots to the pan, and cook briefly over the heat.

2 Pour in 1 litre of boiling water from the kettle, stir in the lentils and stock cube then cover the pan and cook over a medium heat for 15 mins until the lentils are tender. Take off the heat and stir in the parsley. Ladle into bowls, and scatter with extra parsley leaves, if you like.

PER SERVING 285 kcals, fat 5g, saturates 1g, carbs 37g, sugars 12g, fibre 8g, protein 13g, salt 1.6g

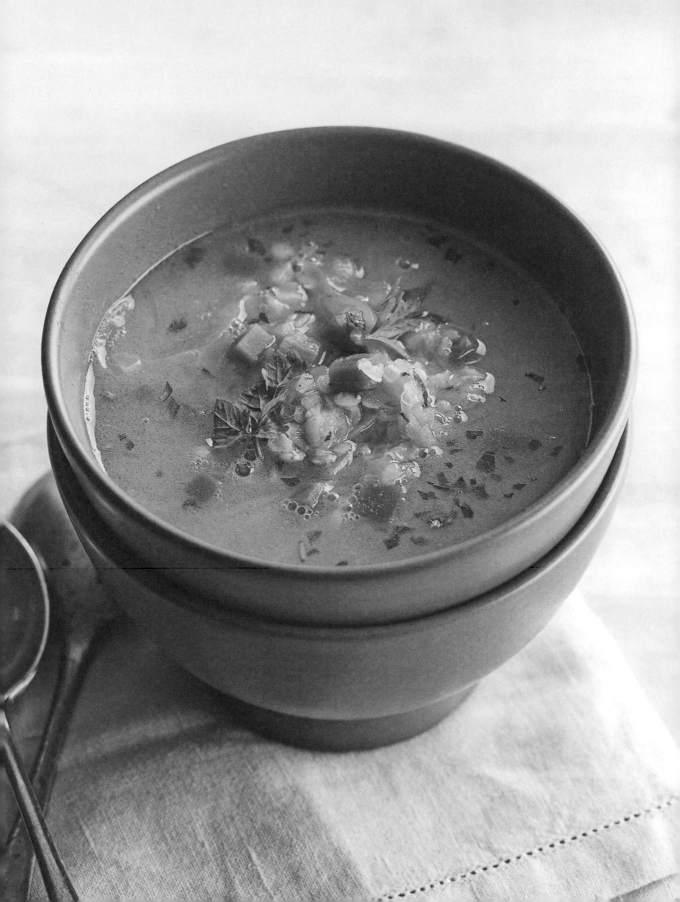

Carrot & Ginger Soup

Low-fat and 3 of your 5 a day, with plenty of fresh ginger for good digestion

🕐 40 mins 🥧 4

- 1 tbsp rapeseed oil
- 1 large onion, chopped
- 2 tbsp coarsely grated ginger
- 2 garlic cloves, sliced
- ½ tsp ground nutmeg, plus a sprinkling
- 850ml/1½ pints vegetable stock
- 500g/1lb 2oz carrots, sliced
- 400g can cannellini beans
- 4 tbsp almonds in their skins, cut into slivers or flaked almonds (optional)

1 Heat the oil in a large pan, add the onion, ginger and garlic and fry for 5 mins until starting to soften. Stir in the nutmeg and cook for a min more.

2 Pour in the stock, add the carrots and beans, including the liquid from the tin, then cover and simmer for 20-25 mins until the carrots are tender.

3 Scoop a third of the mixture into a bowl then blitz the remainder with a hand blender or in a food processor until smooth. Return the reserved soup mixture and heat until bubbling. Serve topped with the almonds and a sprinkle of nutmeg, if you like.

PER SERVING 293 kcals, fat 12g, saturates 1g, carbs 31g, sugars 19g, fibre 8g, protein 10g, salt 0.9g

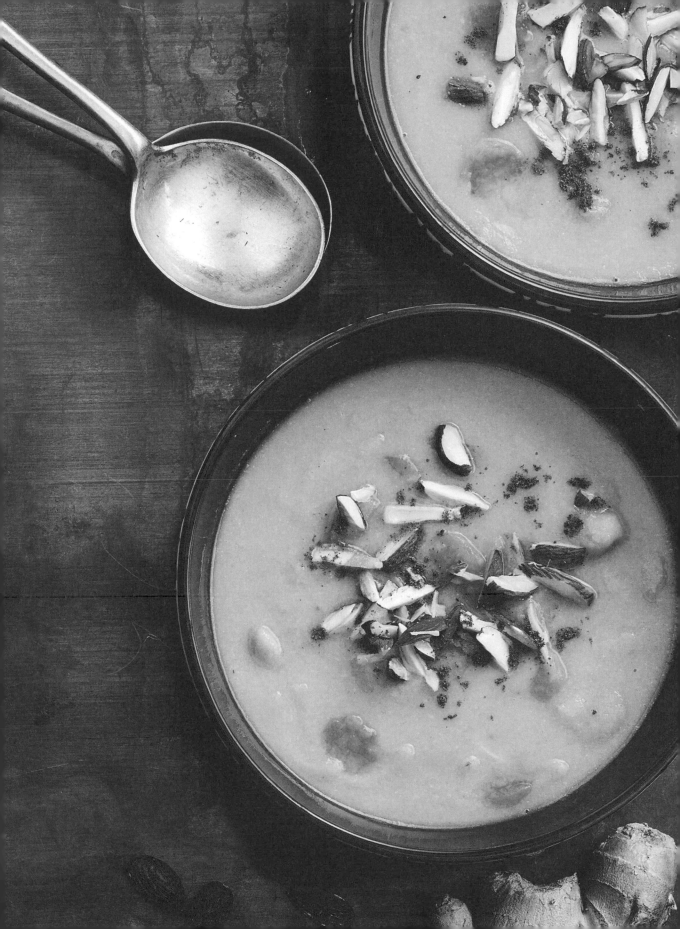

Real Tomato Soup

This so easy to make using store cupboard ingredients. If you have some fresh basil in the fridge or a growing pot, add a handful of leaves, too.

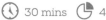 30 mins 4

- 2 tbsp rapeseed or olive oil
- 1 onion, chopped
- 1 garlic clove, finely chopped
- 1 tbsp tomato purée
- 400g can chopped tomatoes
- handful basil leaves (optional, but worth it)
- pinch bicarbonate of soda
- 600ml/1 pint milk

1 Heat the oil in a large pan, then tip in the onion and garlic. Cook over a moderate heat until the onion has softened, about 5 mins. Stir in the tomato purée, then pour in the chopped tomatoes and add the basil leaves, if using, and bring up to the boil. Turn the heat down and leave to simmer for about 15 mins until thick and full of flavour. If you like a smooth soup, whizz the mixture at this point with a hand-held blender.

2 To finish the soup, tip the tomato mixture into a pan. Spoon the bicarbonate of soda into a small bowl and pour over 1 tbsp or so of the milk. Mix together until there are no lumps, then tip into the tomato mix and pour over the milk. Bring up to a boil (the mixture will froth, but don't worry – it will go away). Gently simmer for about 5 mins until ready to serve.

PER SERVING 151 kcals, fat 2g, saturates 2g, carbs 13g, sugars 11g, fibre 11g, protein 7g, salt 0.5g

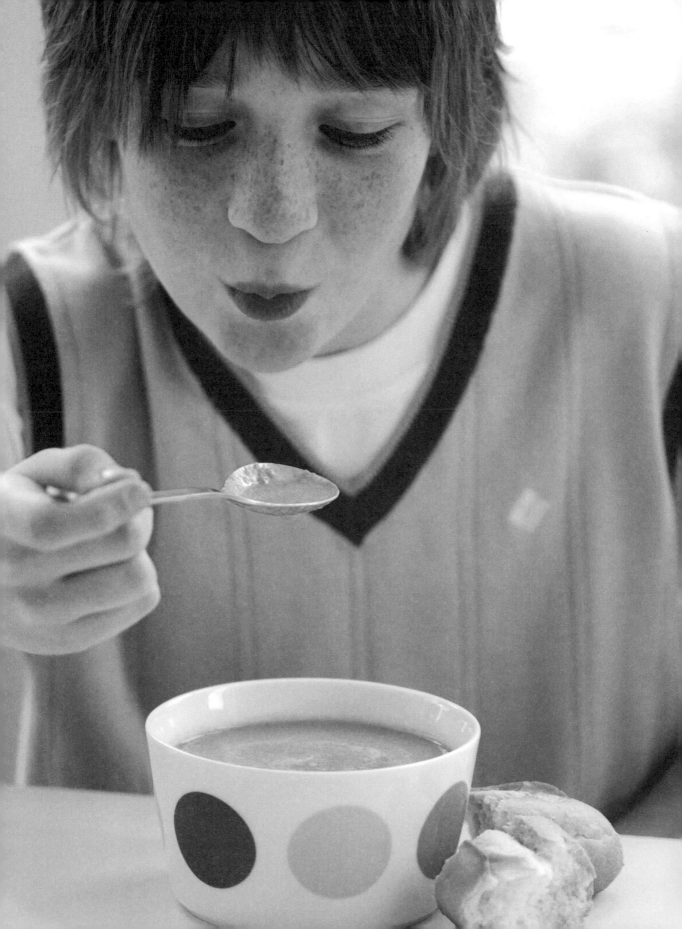

Chunky Butternut Mulligatawny

Chunky, filling and packed full of flavour, yet this is low in fat and calories too.

🕐 1 hour 5 mins 🍽 6

- 2 tbsp olive or rapeseed oil
- 2 onions, finely chopped
- 2 dessert apples, peeled and finely chopped
- 3 celery sticks, finely chopped
- ½ small butternut squash, peeled, seeds removed, chopped into small pieces
- 2 heaped tbsp Madras curry paste
- 1 tbsp ground cinnamon
- 1 tbsp nigella seeds (also called black onion or kalonji seeds) (optional)
- 2 x 400g cans chopped tomatoes
- 1.5 litres/2½ pints vegetable stock
- 140g/5oz brown basmati rice
- small pack parsley, chopped (optional)
- 3 tbsp mango chutney, plus a little to serve (optional)
- natural yogurt, to serve

1 Heat the oil in your largest saucepan. Add the onions, apples and celery with a pinch of salt. Cook for 10 mins, stirring now and then, until softened. Add the butternut squash, curry paste, cinnamon, nigella seeds and a grind of black pepper. Cook for 1 min more, then stir in the tomatoes and stock. Cover with a lid and simmer for 15 mins.

2 By now the vegetables should be tender but not mushy. Stir in the rice, pop the lid back on and simmer for another 12 mins until the rice is cooked through. Taste and add more seasoning if needed. Stir through the parsley and mango chutney, then serve in bowls with yogurt and extra mango chutney on top, if you like.

PER SERVING 212 kcals, fat 5g, saturates 1g, carbs 37g, sugars 15g, fibre 6g, protein 6g, salt 0.5g

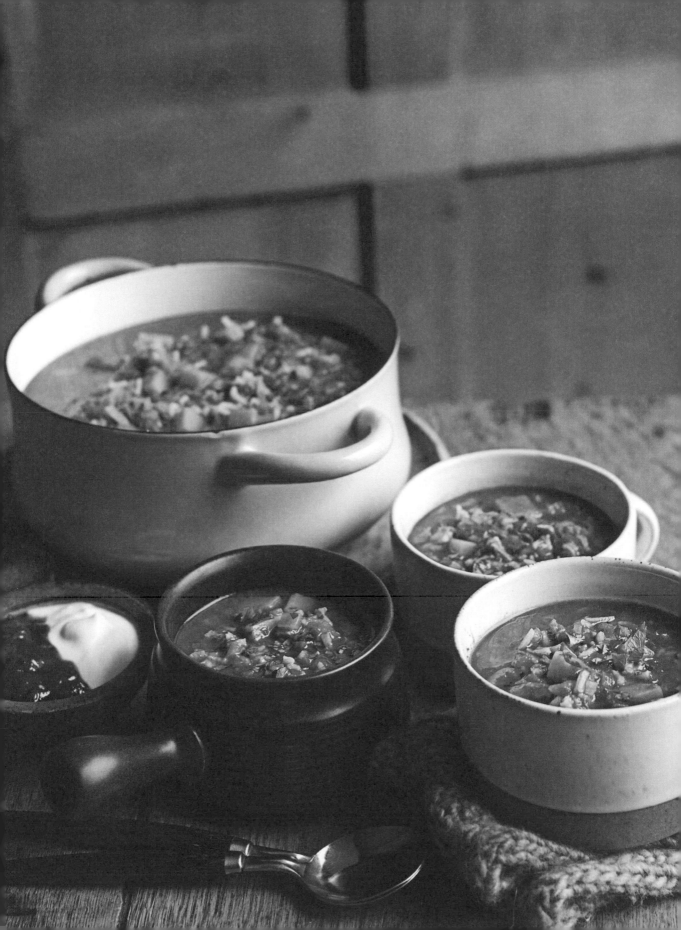

Chunky Mediterranean Tomato Soup

Frozen vegetables are ideal for this soup and will cut down on prep when you are in a hurry.

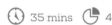 35 mins 4

- 400g/14oz frozen grilled vegetable mix (peppers, aubergine, onions, courgettes)
- 2 tbsp chopped garlic
- handful basil leaves
- 400g can chopped tomatoes
- 1 vegetable stock cube
- 50g/2oz ricotta or low-fat soft cheese per person, beaten with snipped chives and basil or a little pesto, spread on a slice of bread, preferably rye

1 Heat a large non-stick pan, tip in half the vegetables and the garlic, and cook, stirring, over a high heat until they start to soften – about 5 mins. Tip in the basil, tomatoes, stock cube and 2 cans of water, then blitz with a hand-held blender to get the mixture as smooth as you can.

2 Add the remaining frozen veg, cover the pan and cook for 15-20 mins more until the veg is tender. Ladle into bowls. Serve with the bread and herby ricotta on the side.

PER SERVING 212 kcals, fat 7g, saturates 4g, carbs 24g, sugars 4g, fibre 6g, protein 11g, salt 1.5g

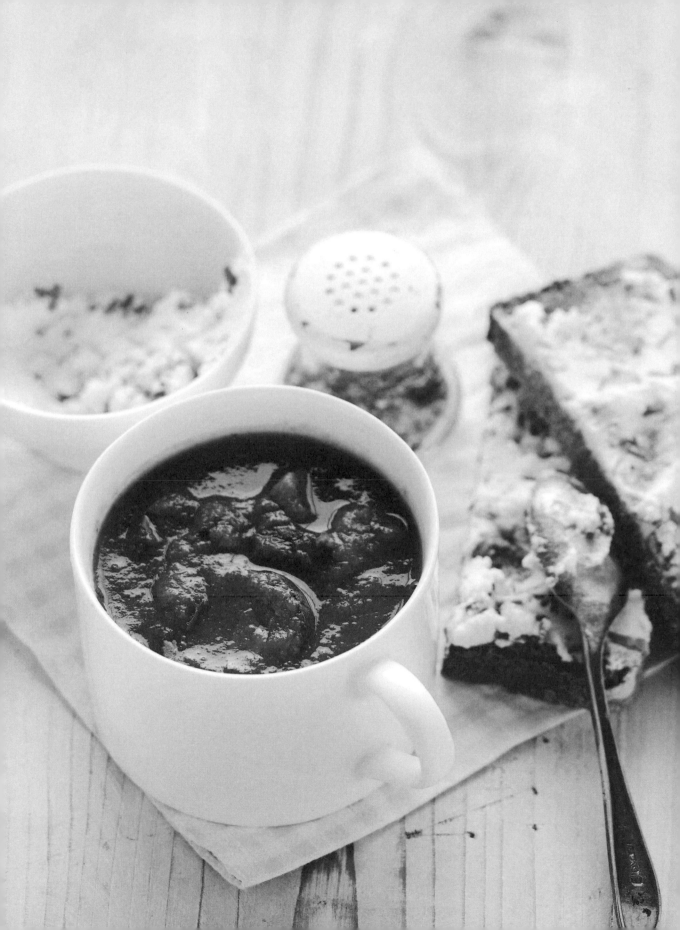

Summer Pistou

This is a cross between a soup and summer vegetable stew, packed with veg and flavoured with aromatic basil. It is low-fat, too.

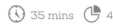 35 mins 4

- 1 tbsp rapeseed oil
- 2 leeks, finely sliced
- 1 large courgette, finely diced
- 1 litre/1¾ pints boiling vegetable stock
- 400g can cannellini or haricot beans, rinsed and drained
- 200g/7oz green beans chopped, fresh or frozen
- 3 tomatoes, chopped
- 3 garlic cloves, chopped
- good handful fresh basil
- 40g/1½oz freshly grated Parmesan

1 Heat the oil in a large pan then fry the leeks and courgette for 5 mins to soften them. Pour in the boiling stock, add three-quarters of the cannellini beans with the green beans and half the tomatoes and simmer for 5-8 mins until the vegetables are all tender.
2 Meanwhile, blitz the remaining tomatoes and beans, garlic and basil in a food processor or in a bowl with a stick blender until smooth then stir in the Parmesan. Stir into the soup, cook for 1 min then ladle into bowls.

PER SERVING 209 kcals, fat 8g, saturates 3g, carbs 18g, sugars 6g, fibre 10g, protein 12g, salt 0.2g

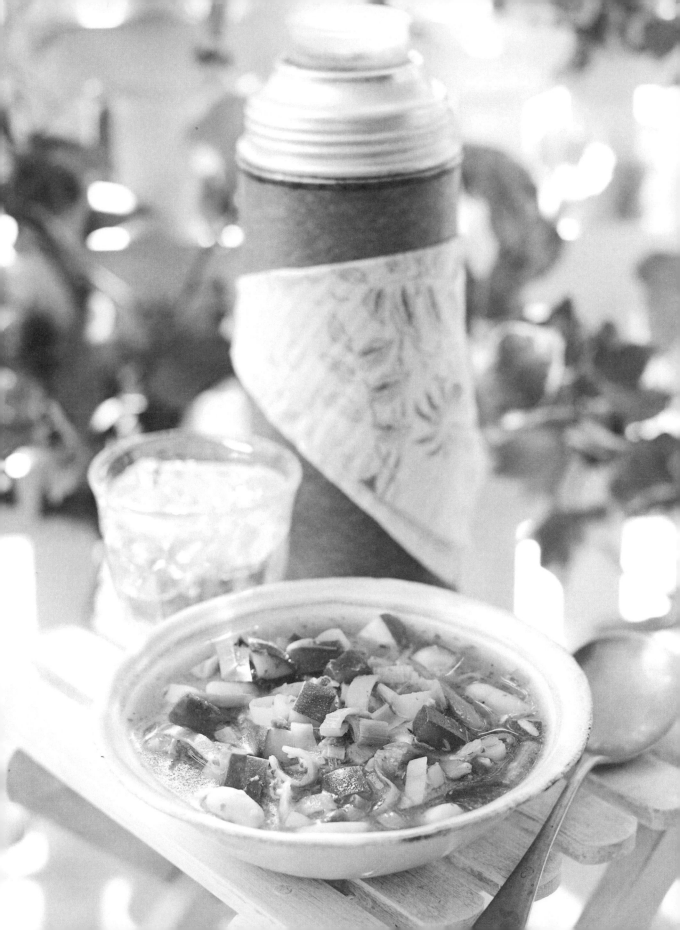

Celeriac & Chorizo Soup

Chorizo is a great ingredient for adding lots of flavour from a relatively small quantity. Celeriac is an under-used vegetable, but if it's not for you, replace it with potato.

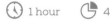 1 hour   4

- 2 tbsp olive oil
- 1 large onion, finely chopped
- 3 garlic cloves, finely chopped
- 6 thyme sprigs, leaves picked or 1 tsp dried
- 600g/1lb 5oz carrots, sliced
- 600g/1lb 5oz celeriac (peeled weight), diced
- 2 litres/3½ pints hot chicken stock
- 140g/5oz chorizo sausage, diced
- ½ tsp smoked paprika

1 Heat the oil in a large saucepan. Add the onion, garlic and thyme then cook on a low heat for 8-10 mins until softened but not coloured. Add the carrots and celeriac and cook for 10 mins more, stirring often. Add the chicken stock and simmer for 20 mins until the vegetables are soft.

2 Blend with a stick blender, then stir in the chorizo and paprika.

PER SERVING 356 kcals, fat 15g, saturates 5g, carbs 21g, sugars 18g, fibre 16g, protein 25g, salt 2.2g

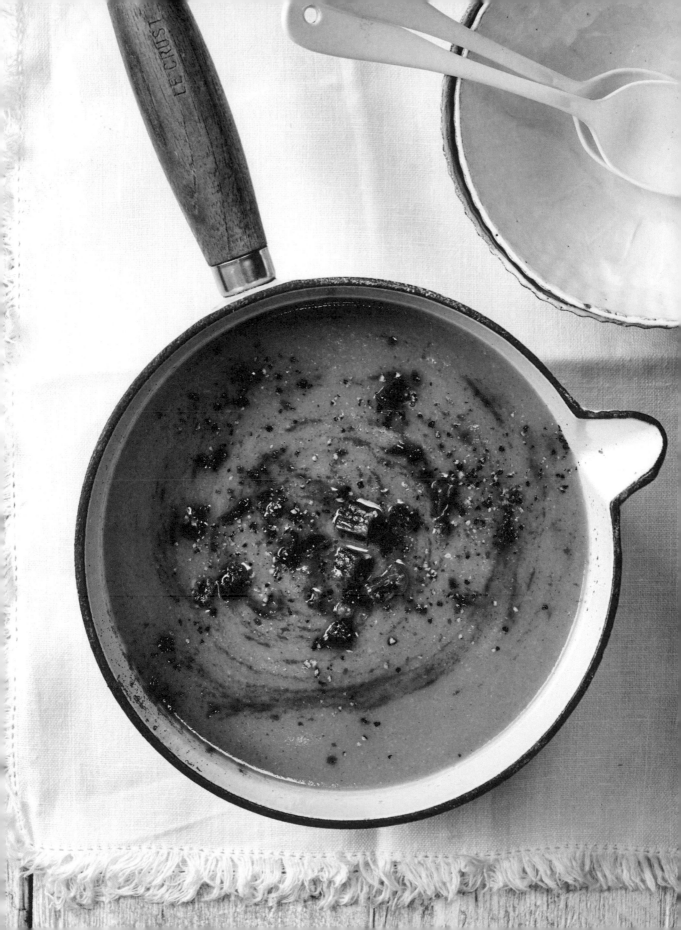

Curried Parsnip Soup

This makes quite a large quantity, but any you don't eat now can easily be frozen ready for a speedy, healthy lunch on another day.

🕐 1 hour   🥧 6-8

- 2 tbsp rapeseed oil
- 3 tbsp Madras curry paste
- 2 onions, roughly chopped
- 500g/1lb 2oz parsnips (around 5 medium parsnips), peeled and cut into chunks
- 140g/5oz red lentils
- 2 Bramley apples peeled, cored and cut into chunks
- 1.5 litres/2¾ pints vegetable stock, made with 1 stock cube
- natural yogurt and chopped coriander, to serve (optional)

1 Heat the oil in a large saucepan. Fry the curry paste and onions together over a medium heat for 3 mins, stirring. Add the parsnips, lentils and apple pieces. Pour over the stock and bring to a simmer. Reduce the heat slightly and cook for 30 mins, stirring occasionally, until the parsnips are very soft and the lentils mushy.

2 Remove from the heat and blitz with a stick blender until smooth (or leave to cool for a few mins, then blend in a food processor). Adjust the seasoning to taste. Heat through gently, then ladle into deep bowls. Serve with natural yogurt and garnish with fresh coriander.

PER SERVING (8) 204 kcals, fat 5g, saturates 1g, carbs 24g, sugars 10g, fibre 8g, protein 12g, salt 0.7g

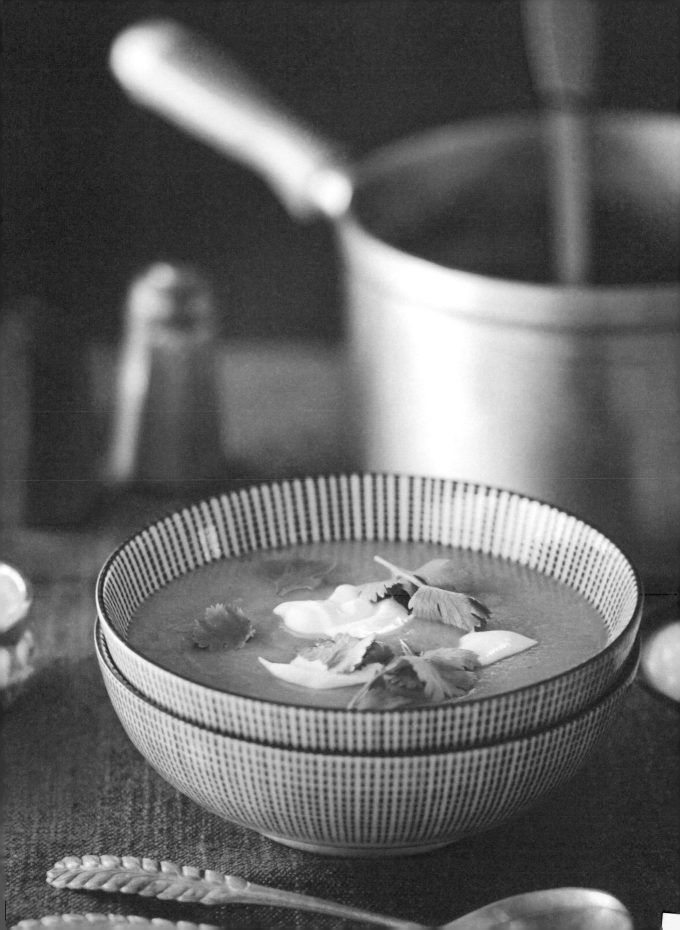

Egg & Rocket Pizzas

If you have any wraps left over from a previous meal, they make a great pizza base.

🕐 25 mins   🥧 2

- 2 tortilla wraps, wholewheat or seeded are best
- a little olive oil, for brushing
- 1 roasted red pepper from a jar
- 2 tomatoes
- 2 tbsp tomato purée
- 1 tbsp chopped dill or basil
- 2 tbsp chopped parsley
- 2 eggs
- 65g pack rocket
- ½ red onion, very thinly sliced

1 Heat oven to 200C/180C fan/gas 6. Lay the tortillas on two baking sheets, brush sparingly with the oil, then bake for 3 mins.
2 Meanwhile, chop the pepper and tomatoes and mix with the tomato purée and herbs. Turn the tortillas over and spread with the tomato mixture, leaving the centre free.
3 Break an egg into the centre of each tortilla then return to the oven for 10 mins or until the eggs are just set and the tortillas are crispy round the edges. Serve scattered with the rocket and onion.

PER SERVING 327 kcals, fat 11g, saturates 3g, carbs 39g, sugars 8g, fibre 5g, protein 15g, salt 1.0g

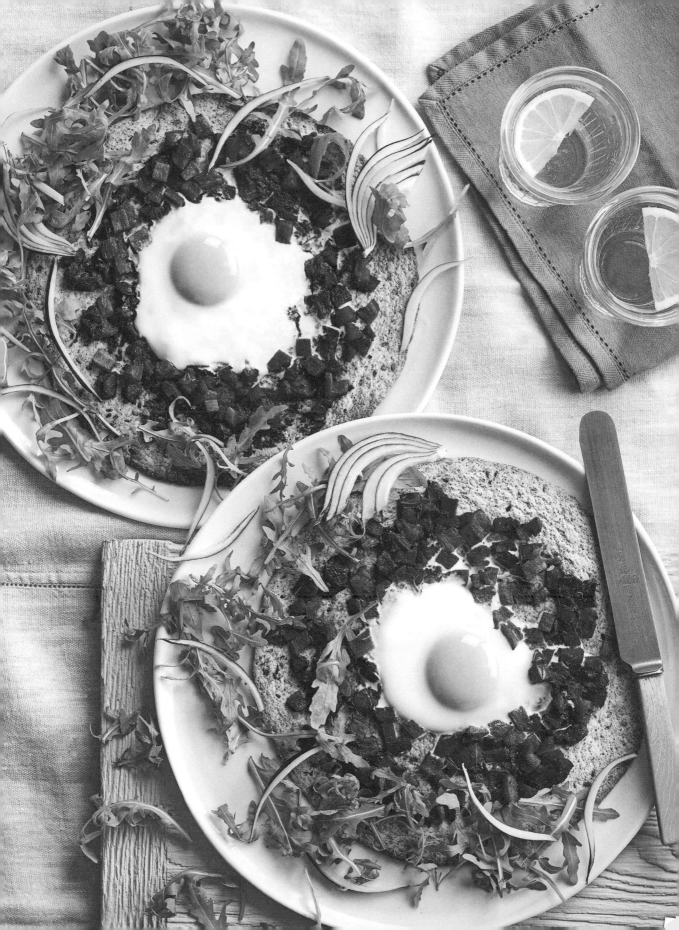

Peanut Butter Paté with Fruit & Veg Sticks

This paté is perfect for spreading on crisp apple slices, celery and carrot sticks and will offer you an amazing 4 of your 5 a day. Add extra liquid if you want a dipping consistency.

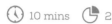 10 mins   2

- 380g can chickpeas
- ½ lemon, zest and juice (use the half of lemon not used to squeeze over the apple to stop it browning, if you like)
- 1 tbsp tahini
- ½-1 tsp smoked paprika
- 2 tbsp roasted, but not salted peanuts
- 1 tsp rapeseed oil
- 2 crisp red skinned apples, cored and cut into slices
- 2 carrots, cut into sticks
- 4 celery sticks, cut into lengths

1 Drain the chickpeas, but retain the liquid. Tip three-quarters of the chickpeas into a food processor and add the lemon zest and juice, tahini, paprika, peanuts and oil with 3 tbsp chickpea liquid. Blitz in a food processor until smooth then stir in the reserved chickpeas. Serve with the fruit and veg sticks.

PER SERVING 336 kcals, fat 16g, saturates 2g, carbs 35g, sugars 16g, fibre 13g, protein 15g, salt 0.8g

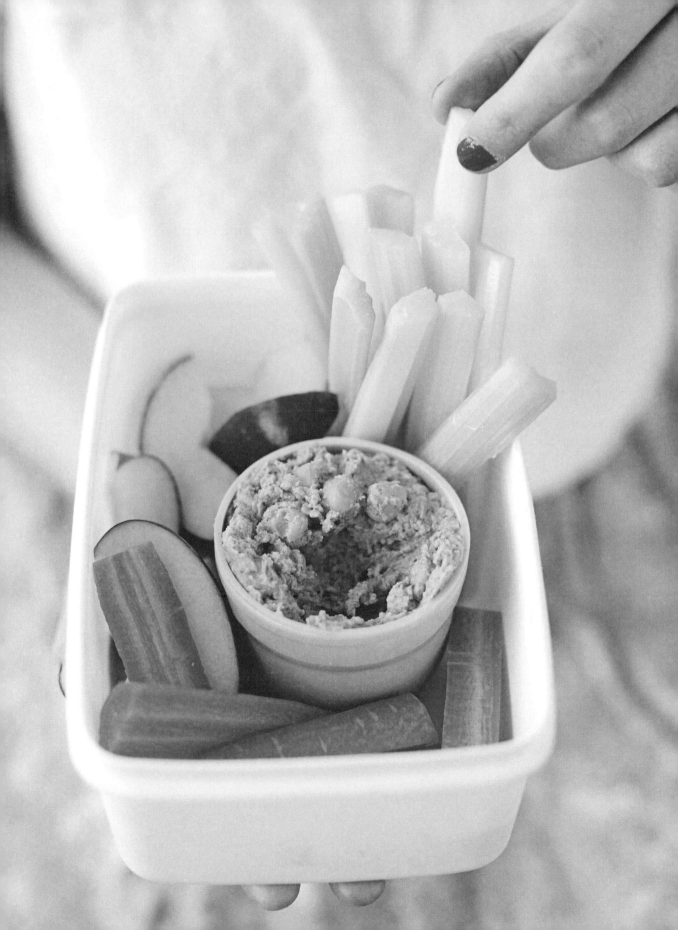

Open Prawn-Cocktail Sandwich

Open sandwiches are a great option if you don't want too much bread. Just pile on the topping for a substantial lunch!

🕐 15 mins   🥧 2

- 2 tbsp light mayonnaise
- 1 tbsp tomato ketchup
- 2 tbsp chopped dill leaves (optional)
- 1 lemon, cut into 8 wedges
- 100g pack cooked and peeled North Atlantic prawns
- ½ cucumber, deseeded and diced
- 2 handfuls cherry tomatoes, halved
- 2 thin slices wholemeal or rye bread
- 25g bag rocket leaves

1 Make the dressing in a medium bowl by mixing together the mayonnaise, ketchup, half the dill, the juice from 4 of the lemon wedges and some seasoning. Toss in the prawns, cucumber and tomatoes.
2 Arrange the bread on two plates, top each with rocket and pile on the prawn filling. Scatter with the remaining dill and serve with the remaining lemon wedges, for squeezing over.

PER SERVING 173 kcals, fat 3g, saturates none, carbs 22g, sugars 7g, fibre 3g, protein 17g salt 1.6g

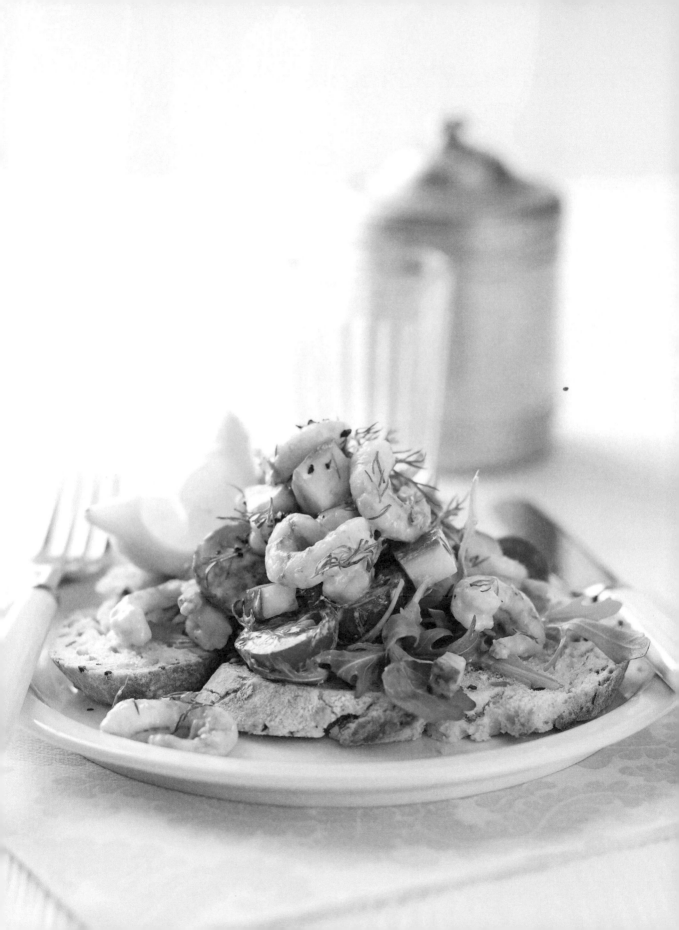

Piri-piri Prawn Flatbreads

This makes a fantastic summer lunch, use tortillas if you can't find flatbreads. If you don't want to griddle the peppers and prawns you can stir-fry them instead.

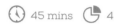 45 mins 4

- 150ml pot soured cream or plain whole yogurt
- juice 1 lemon
- small pack mint, finely chopped
- 300g/11oz peeled raw prawns
- 4 tsp rapeseed oil
- 3 large garlic cloves, crushed
- 1 red chilli, deseeded and finely chopped
- 1 tsp smoked paprika
- 4 large flatbreads or tortillas
- 3 red peppers, deseeded and thinly sliced
- 3 Little Gem lettuces, shredded

1 Heat oven to 160C/140C fan/gas 3. Mix the soured cream or yogurt with 1 tbsp lemon juice, the mint and seasoning, cover and put in the fridge. Toss the prawns in 2 tsp oil, 1 tbsp lemon juice, the garlic, chilli and paprika. Wrap the breads in foil and put in the oven to warm.

2 Heat a griddle pan on a medium-high heat. Toss the peppers in the remaining 2 tsp oil, and cook on the griddle for 5-10 mins until charred and softened (you may need to do this in two batches). Keep warm in the oven while you cook the prawns on the griddle pan for 2-3 mins each side until pink, cooked through and lightly charred. Serve with the warm flatbreads or tortillas, lettuce, peppers and soured cream or yogurt.

PER SERVING 437 kcals, fat 13g, saturates 6g, carbs 51g, sugars 13g, fibre 6g, protein 25g, salt 1.2g

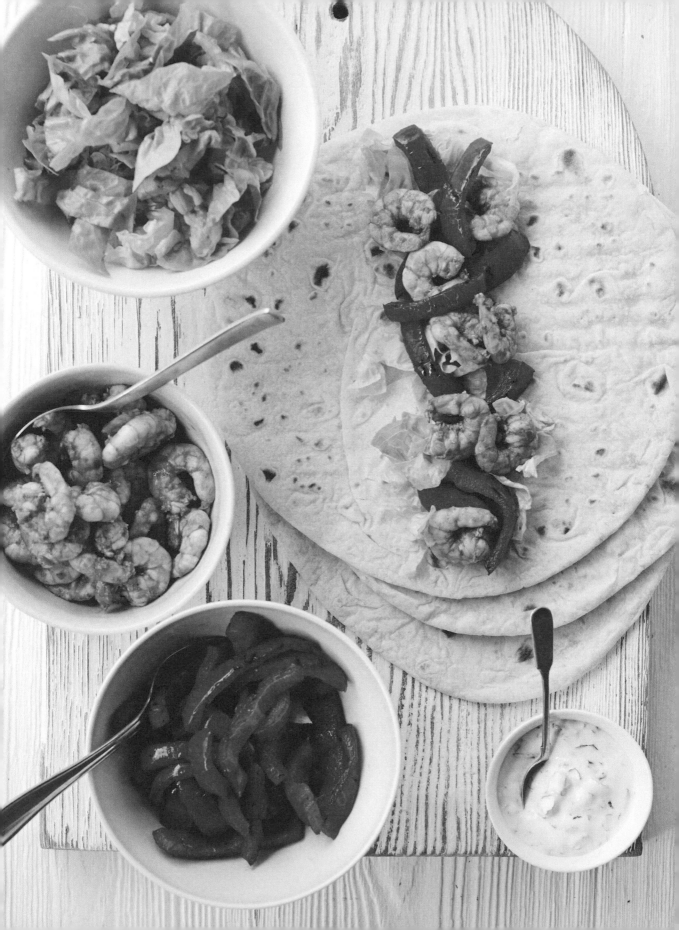

Spicy Chicken & Avocado Wraps

Lean chicken breast is a great source of low-fat protein and one breast can easily serve two when combined with veg.

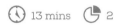 13 mins   2

- 1 large skinless chicken breast
- generous squeeze juice from ½ lime
- ½ tsp mild chilli powder
- 1 garlic clove, chopped
- 2 tsp olive oil
- 2 wraps, seeded or wholewheat
- 1 avocado, halved and stoned
- 1 roast red pepper from a jar, sliced
- few sprigs coriander, chopped

1 Thinly slice the chicken at an angle so you end up with quite large pieces of chicken then mix with the lime juice, chilli powder and garlic.
2 Heat the oil in a non-stick frying pan then fry the chicken for a couple of mins – it will cook very quickly so keep an eye on it. Meanwhile warm the wraps according to the pack instructions or if you have a gas hob, heat them over the flame to slightly char them.
3 Squash half an avocado onto each wrap, add the peppers to the pan to warm them through then pile onto the wraps and sprinkle over the coriander. Roll up, cut in half and eat with your fingers.

PER SERVING 403 kcals, fat 16g, saturates 4g, carbs 32g, sugars 2g, fibre 5g, protein 29g, salt 0.8g

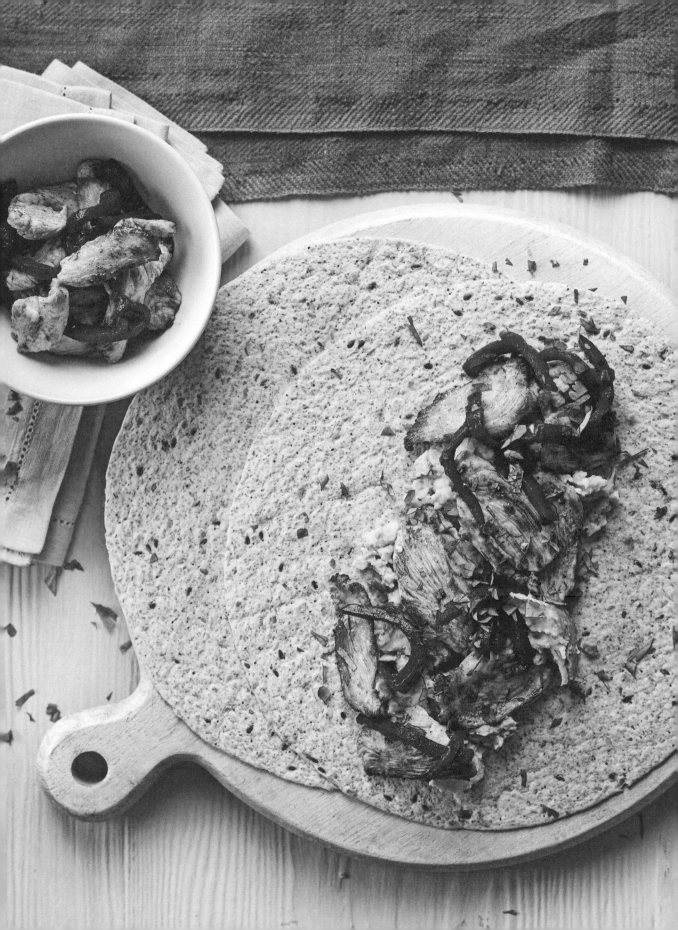

Carrot & Houmous Roll-ups

Keep a pack of wraps in the storecupboard and a quick snack is never far away. This is a good idea for a healthy packed lunch to take to work.

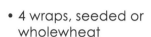 10 mins 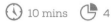 4

- 4 wraps, seeded or wholewheat
- 200g tub houmous
- 4 carrots, grated
- handful of rocket leaves

1 Lay the wraps on a board and spread with the houmous.
2 Scatter with the carrots and rocket then roll up and eat.

PER SERVING 355 kcals, fat 19g, saturates 3g, carbs 37g, sugars 8g, fibre 6g, protein 10g, salt 1.09g

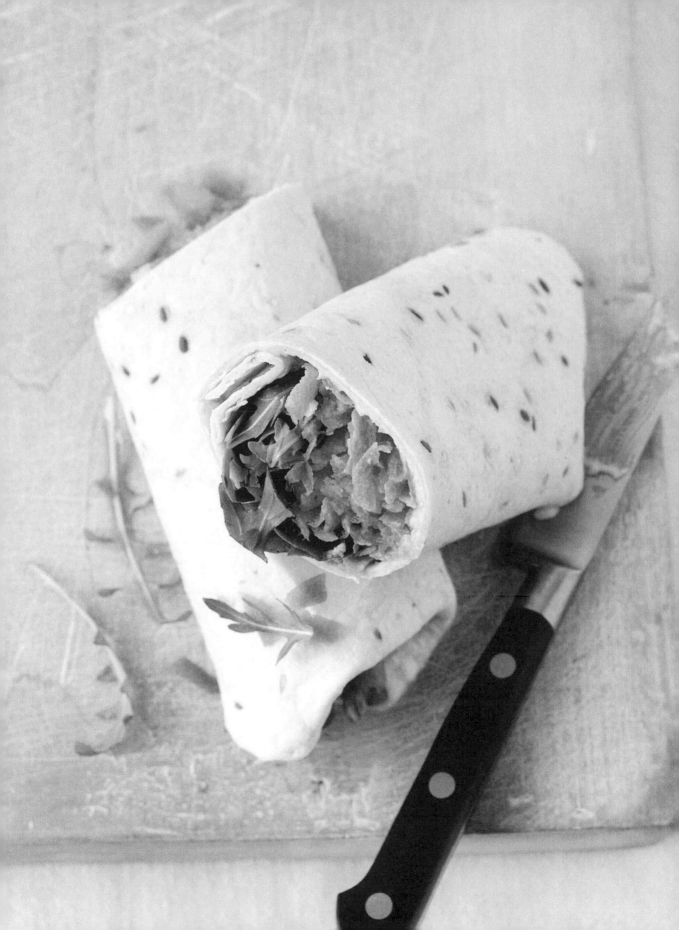

Stuffed Avocado with Spicy Beans & Feta

Avocados are well worth including in your diet for their healthy oils. Their creamy nature means there's no need for oil in the dressing, just the refreshing zing of lime.

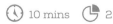 10 mins   2

- ½ tsp cumin seeds
- 210g can red kidney beans, rinsed and drained
- grated zest and juice of ½ large lime, plus wedges
- 3 tomatoes, diced
- 1 small red onion, finely chopped
- 1 green chilli, deseeded and finely chopped
- handful fresh coriander, chopped, plus a few extra leaves
- 85g/3oz feta cheese, goat's, ewe's or reduced fat
- 1 large or 2 small avocados, stoned and halved

1 Put the cumin seeds in a small pan and lightly toast over the heat. Tip into a large bowl and mix with the beans, lime zest and juice, tomatoes, onion, chilli and coriander. Crumble in the feta and gently toss.
2 Serve on top of the avocado halves, scattering with a few extra coriander leaves and squeezing over a little extra lime from the wedges.

PER SERVING 411 kcals, fat 29g, saturates 10g, carbs 18g, sugars 7g, fibre 12g, protein 32g, salt 2g

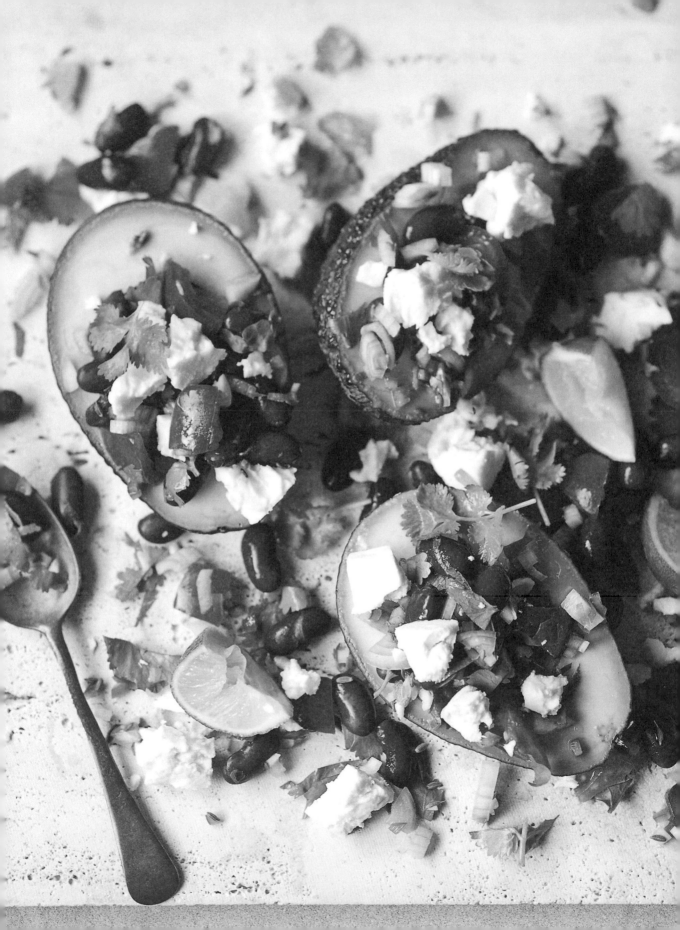

Falafel Burgers

Whizz up chickpeas with garlic, spices and herbs to make delicious vegetarian burger that's filling, too.

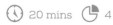 20 mins · 4

- 250g/9oz chickpeas from a can
- 1 medium onion, finely chopped
- 2 garlic cloves, crushed
- 2 tsp ground coriander
- 2 tsp ground cumin
- small pack flat-leaf parsley, chopped
- 2 rounded tbsp plain flour
- 2 tbsp rapeseed oil
- 100g/4oz houmous
- 4 burger buns, preferably wholewheat, cut in half
- watercress or salad, to serve

1 Drain, rinse and dry the chickpeas thoroughly, then tip into the bowl of a food processor. Pulse until lightly broken up into coarse crumbs.

2 Add the onion, garlic, spices, parsley, flour and some seasoning, and continue to pulse until combined. Using your hands, gently form the mixture into 4 patties about 10cm in diameter and 2cm thick.

3 In a large pan, heat the oil and fry the falafels on each side for 2-3 mins or until golden (you may need to do this in batches). Lightly griddle the burger buns on the cut side in a griddle pan, or toast under the grill.

4 Spread one side of each bun with houmous, top with a falafel burger, add a handful of watercress or salad, then pop the remaining bun half on top.

PER SERVING 476 kcals, fat 15g, saturates 2g, carbs 63g, sugars 5g, fibre 7g, protein 17g, salt 2.0g

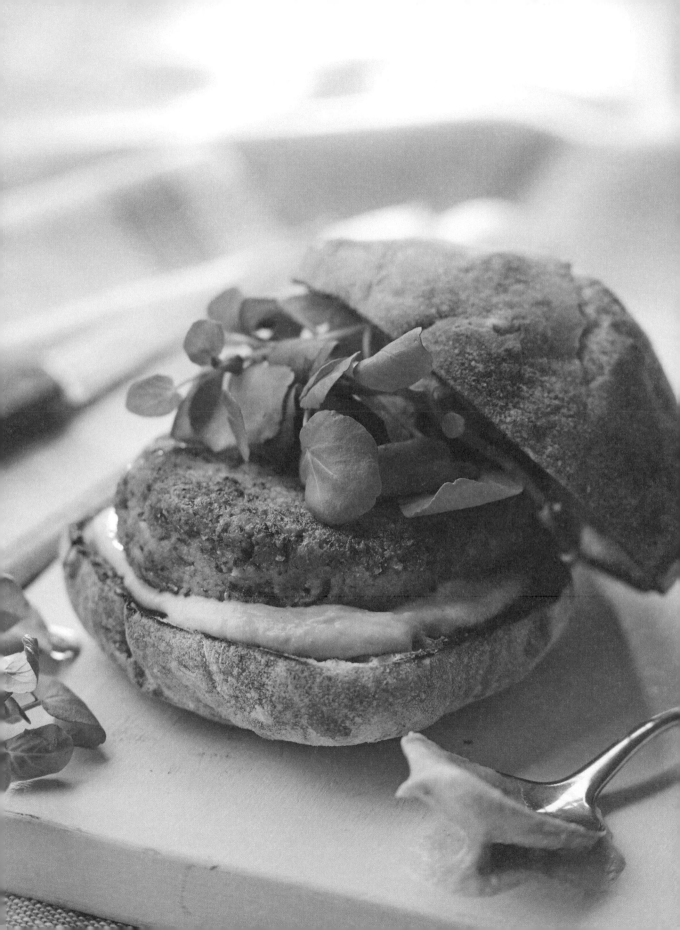

Rainbow Orzo Salad

Orzo is a variety of pasta, the size of rice and fantastic for lunch boxes mixed with other ingredients. You could use snapped spaghetti instead, or another small pasta shape.

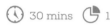 30 mins · 1

- 2 peppers, any colour, deseeded and sliced
- 1 red onion, cut into thin wedges
- 1 tbsp olive oil
- 6 cherry tomatoes, halved
- 25g/1oz orzo pasta
- 25g/1oz feta, crumbled
- 2 tbsp roughly chopped basil

1 Heat oven to 200C/180C fan/gas 6. Put the peppers and onion in a roasting tin and drizzle with half the oil. Roast for 20 mins, adding the tomatoes for the final 5 mins. Leave to cool.

2 Cook the orzo following the pack instructions, then run under cold water to cool before draining thoroughly. Toss with the vegetables, the remaining oil, the feta and basil.

PER SERVING 422 kcals, fat 18g, saturates 6g, carbs 52g, sugars 30g, fibre 9g, protein 13g, salt 1g

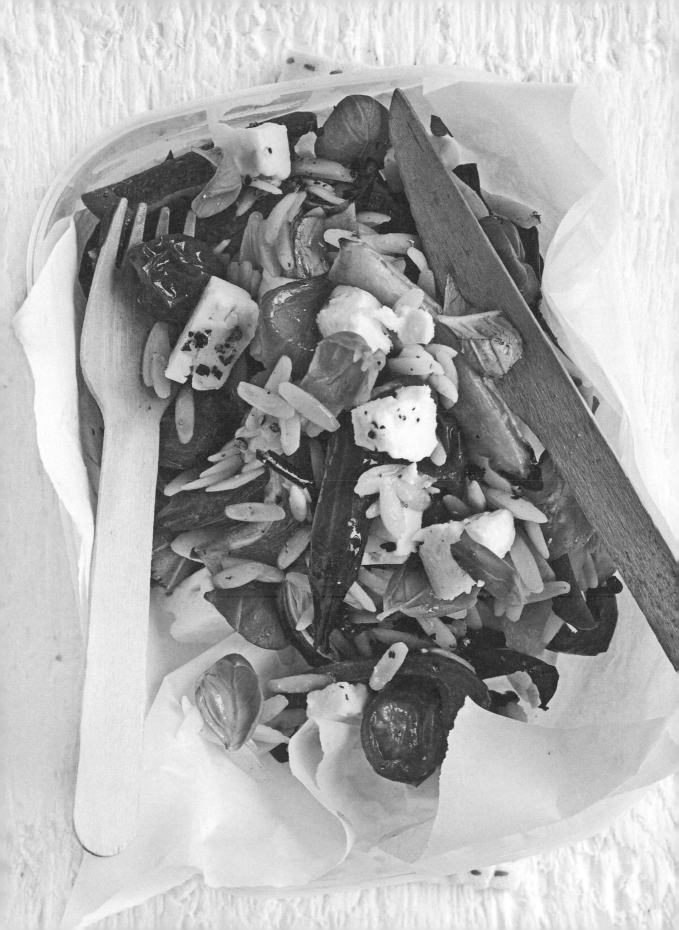

Courgette, Broccoli & Gremolata Pasta

Fresh broccoli, well known as a 'superfood' as it is packed with antioxidants, takes a star roll in this summery pasta dish, which is boosted with vitamin C from the parsley and lemon.

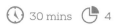 30 mins 4

- 3 garlic cloves, finely grated
- zest of 2 lemons, plus a squeeze of juice
- small bunch of parsley, finely chopped
- 200g/7oz broccoli, broken into florets
- 400g/14oz pasta bows or other shapes, preferably wholewheat
- 1 tsp olive oil
- 2 courgettes, chopped

1 To make the gremolata, mix the garlic, lemon zest and juice in a small bowl with the parsley and some seasoning.
2 Bring a large pan of water to the boil, add the broccoli and cook for 2–3 mins until just tender. Use a slotted spoon to remove, then set aside. Bring the water back to the boil, add the pasta and cook according to the pack instructions.
3 Heat the olive oil in a frying pan, add the courgettes and cook over a high heat until starting to turn golden, tip in the broccoli and continue to cook until warmed through.
4 Drain the pasta, reserving about 2 tablespoons of the cooking water, then add the pasta, cooking water and gremolata to the vegetables. Mix well and serve.

PER SERVING 390 kcals, fat 4g, saturates 1g, carbs 79g, sugars 4g, fibre 5g, protein 16g, salt 0.04g

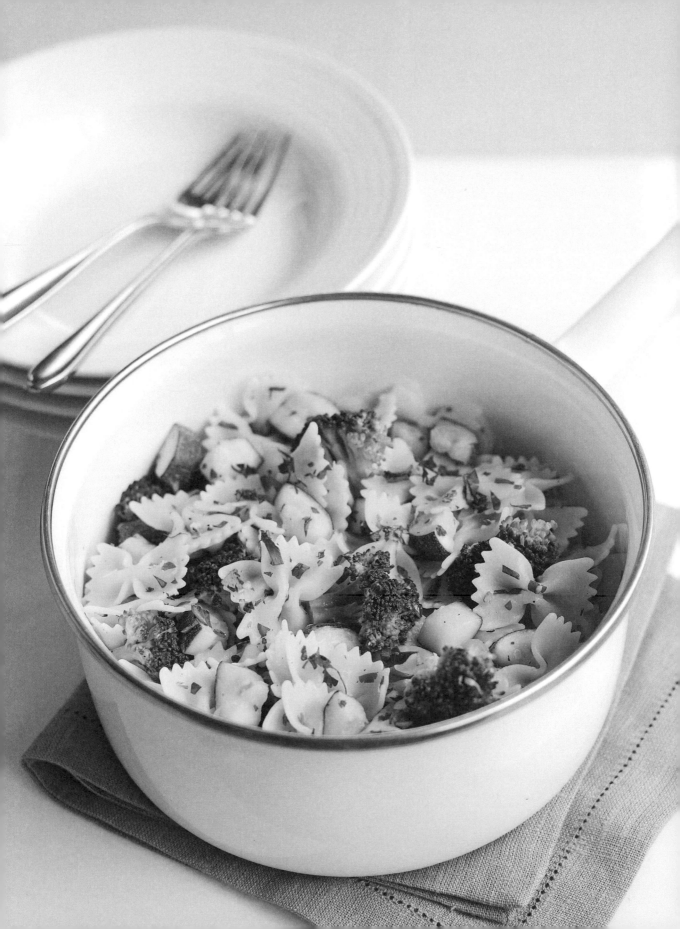

Spiced Pea & Potato Rolls

Children will love these crispy, crunchy spring rolls, and as they are packed with veg, they're a healthy choice for a lunchtime snack. It is a delicious way of using up leftover veg, too.

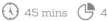 45 mins 4

- 2 tbsp rapeseed oil
- 2 onions, finely sliced
- 300g/10oz potatoes, cut into small cubes
- 1 heaped tbsp Madras curry paste
- 140g/5oz frozen peas
- 4 large sheets filo pastry, cut in half
- tomato and onion salad and mango chutney, to serve

1 Heat oven to 220C/200C fan/gas 7. Heat half the oil in a non-stick frying pan. Tip in the onions and cook until soft and golden.

2 Meanwhile, boil the potatoes for 5 mins, until tender, then drain. Tip into the onions and fry for 2 mins. Stir in the curry paste and cook for 2 mins. Add the peas, plus 1 tbsp water. Cook for 1 min then cool slightly.

3 Brush half the filo half-sheets with some of the remaining oil, then lay the remaining sheets on top so you have four double layers. Spoon a quarter of the potato mix along one edge of each, leaving space at each end. Fold in the ends then roll up to seal. Put seam-side down on a baking sheet, brush with the remaining oil and bake for 20 mins or until crisp. Serve warm with mango chutney and a tomato and onion salad.

PER SERVING 240 kcals, fat 8g, saturates 1g, carbs 37g, sugars 6g, fibre 4g, protein 7g, salt 0.46g

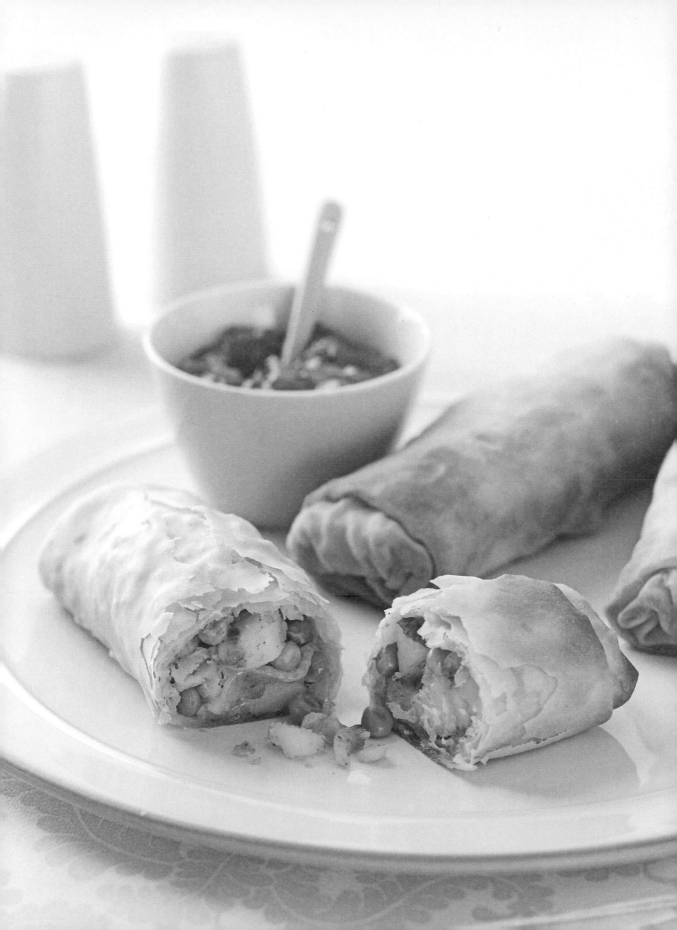

Italian Stuffed Sweet Peppers

Take five ingredients and whip up this simple midweek supper. You can save time and use halved roasted peppers from a jar then start the recipe from step 2 if you like.

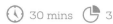 30 mins   3

- 3 red peppers, Romano if you like, halved and deseeded
- 160g pack semi-dried tomatoes and mozzarella balls in olive oil
- 140g/5oz couscous, preferably wholewheat
- 2 tbsp pesto
- 5 tbsp dried breadcrumbs

1 Heat oven to 200C/180C fan/gas 6. Arrange the peppers, cut-side up, on a baking tray. Brush with a little oil from the pack of tomatoes and mozzarella, then season. Cook for 10 mins to soften slightly.

2 Meanwhile, mix the couscous in a bowl with the pesto and pour over 125ml boiling water. Cover and leave for 5 mins to fluff up. Drain the tomatoes and mozzarella well, then mix into the couscous. Divide between the peppers, then sprinkle over the breadcrumbs.

3 Bake for 15-20 mins until the top is crisp and the peppers are tender.

PER SERVING 419 kcals, fat 11g, saturates 2g, carbs 58g, sugars 9g, fibre 6g, protein 15g, salt 0.8g

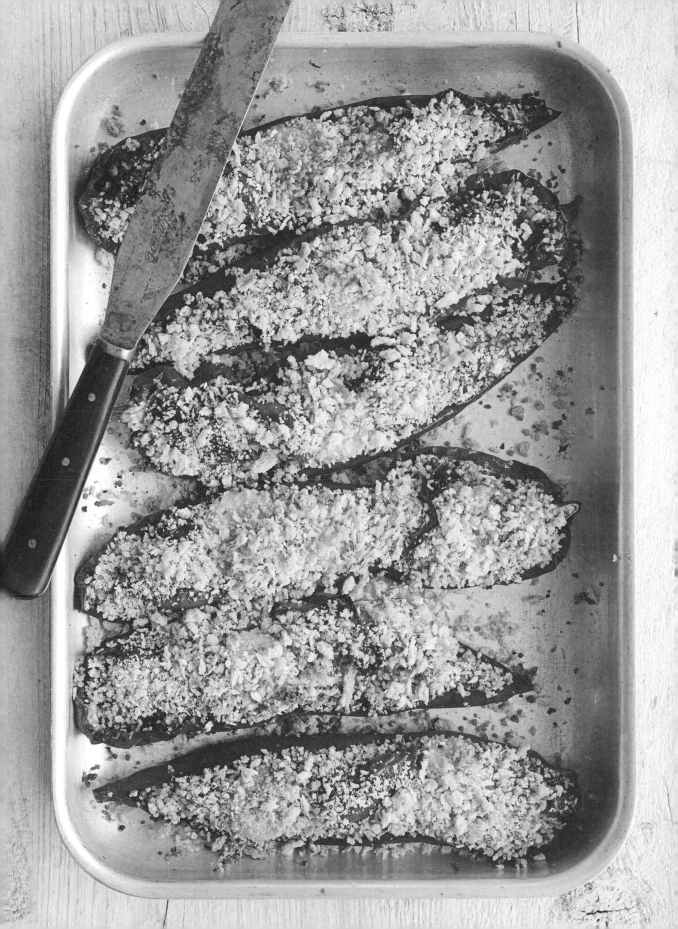

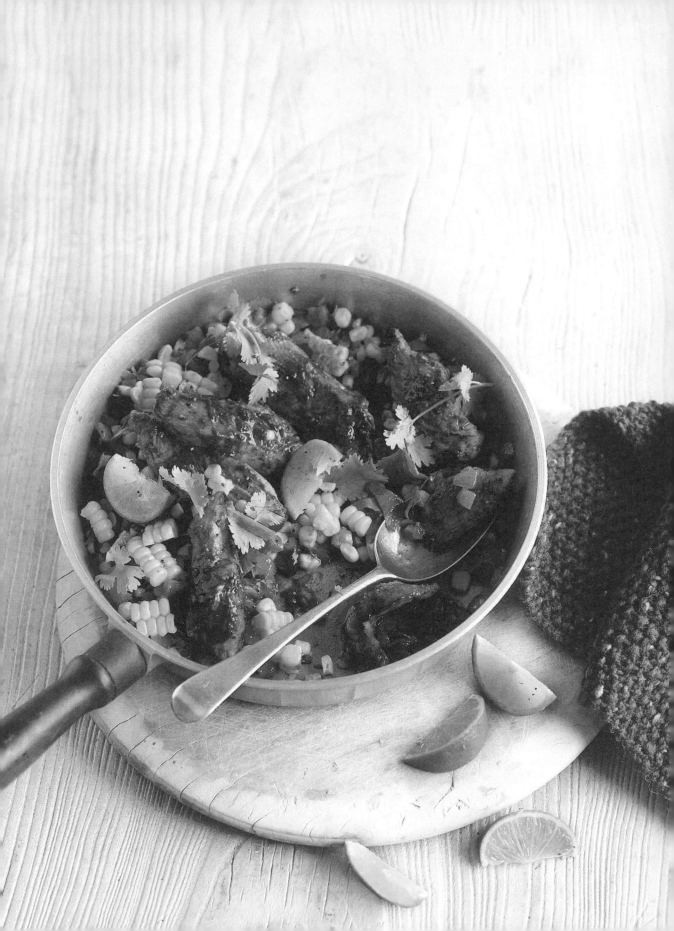

Chapter 3:

CHICKEN & MEAT SUPPERS

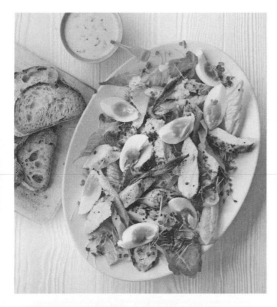

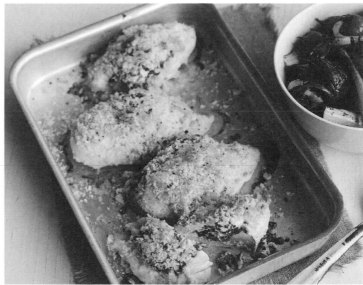

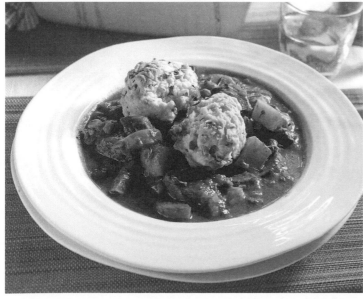

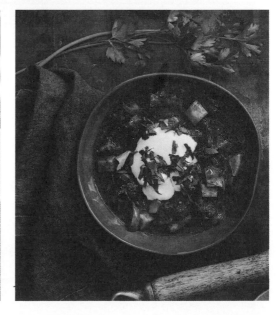

Chinese Poached Chicken

This makes a lovely light Asian-inspired supper to serve with rice. If you have broth leftover, you can make a simple soup by adding some noodles as you reheat it.

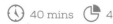 40 mins 4

- large piece of ginger, 1 tbsp finely grated, the rest sliced
- 3 garlic cloves
- 1 tsp black peppercorns
- few pinches Chinese 5 spice (optional)
- 1 tbsp soy sauce, preferably reduced-salt, plus 2–3 tsp (optional)
- 4 chicken legs
- 3 tbsp sesame oil
- 2 bunches spring onions, chopped
- 4 pak choi, halved or a few Chinese leaves thickly sliced
- cooked long grain or brown rice, to serve

1 Put the sliced ginger, the garlic, peppercorns, Chinese spice, if using, and half the soy in a large pan with the chicken legs. Add enough water to cover. Bring to the boil, then reduce to a low simmer, put on the lid and poach for 30 mins.
2 Meanwhile, heat a pan and add the sesame oil and spring onions. Soften for 1 min, then remove from the heat and stir in the grated ginger and remaining soy sauce to make a relish.
3 When the chicken is ready, remove from the pan. Add the pak choi to the poaching liquid and cook for 3–4 mins. Strain the poaching liquid to remove the ginger, garlic and peppercorns, reserving the liquid. Pull the skin from the chicken legs and discard. Tear the meat into thick pieces. Serve in bowls with rice, the pak choi, a ladle of the hot chicken broth, the spring onion relish and extra soy sauce, if you like.

PER SERVING 317 kcals, fat 20g, saturates 5g, carbs 4g, sugars 3g, fibre 3g, protein 30g, salt 1.1g

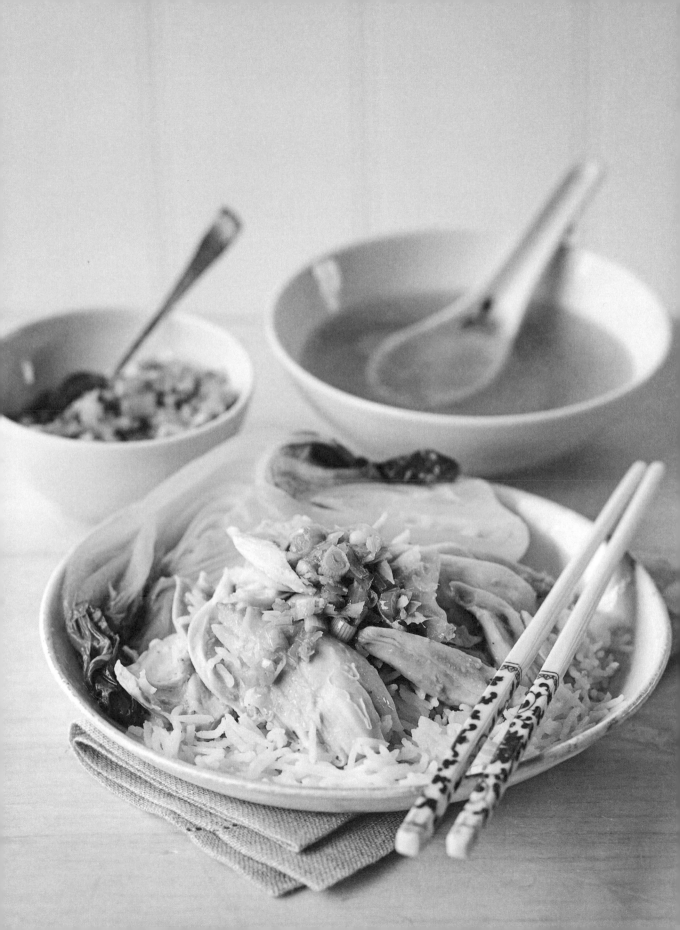

Skinny Chicken Caesar Salad

This high-protein, low-fat salad is loosely based on the American classic.

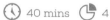 40 mins 4

- 4 skinless chicken breasts
- 2 tsp olive oil
- juice 1 lemon
- 1 large romaine or cos lettuce, chopped into large pieces
- 1 punnet salad cress
- 4 hard-boiled eggs, peeled and quartered
- 25g/1oz Parmesan, finely grated
- 50g/2oz anchovy fillets, half chopped, half left whole
- 170g pot fat-free Greek yogurt

1 Put the chicken breasts in a large bowl with the olive oil and 1 tbsp lemon juice. Heat the grill to high. Put the chicken breasts on a foil-lined baking tray and cook under the grill for 10–12 mins until cooked through, turning once during cooking. Transfer to a plate or board and rest for 5 mins then slice.

2 Arrange the lettuce, cress and eggs on a platter or serving plates and top with the sliced chicken. Mix together the Parmesan, chopped anchovies, yogurt and remaining lemon juice, and pour over the salad. Arrange the whole anchovy fillets on top of each salad.

PER SERVING 321 kcals, fat 12g, saturates 4g, carbs 4g, sugars 3g, fibre 3g, protein 48g, salt 1.8g

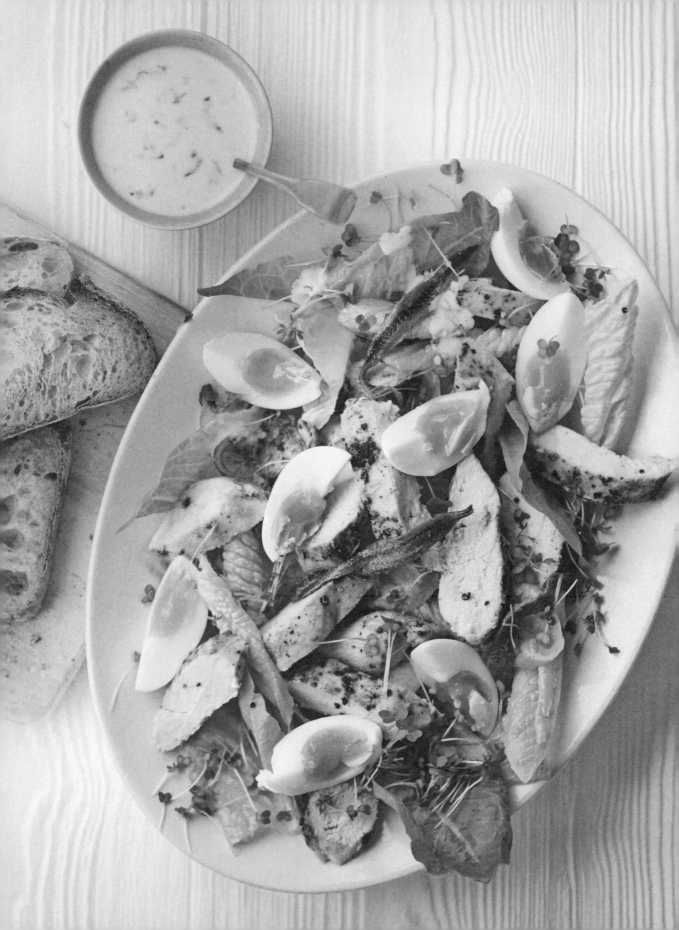

Fruity Caribbean Curry

Kidney beans, pineapple and veg, notch up 4 of your 5 a day and make chicken drumsticks go further in this sweet and hot family curry.

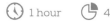 1 hour 4

- 2 tsp rapeseed oil
- 4 chicken drumsticks, skin removed
- 2 large red onions, chopped
- 2 peppers (any colours will do), deseeded and chopped
- 3–4 tbsp mild curry powder or Madras curry paste
- 425g can pineapple chunks in unsweetened juice
- 400g can coconut milk
- 400g can kidney beans, drained
- 2–4 tbsp hot pepper sauce (depending on how hot you like it)
- small bunch coriander, chopped, to serve
- rice, to serve, preferably brown (optional)

1 Heat the oil in a large frying pan. Add the chicken and brown well on all sides, then transfer to a plate. Add the onions and peppers to the pan, and cook for 5 mins until the veg starts to soften. Return the chicken to the pan and add the curry powder or paste, then tip in the pineapple with its juice, and the coconut milk. Simmer, uncovered, for 40 mins until the chicken is tender and the sauce has reduced and thickened a little.

2 Add the beans and pepper sauce to the pan. Simmer for another 2–3 mins until the beans are warmed through, then scatter with coriander and serve with rice.

PER SERVING 458 kcals, fat 23g, saturates 16g, carbs 36g, sugars 23g, fibre 11g, protein 21g, salt 1.5g

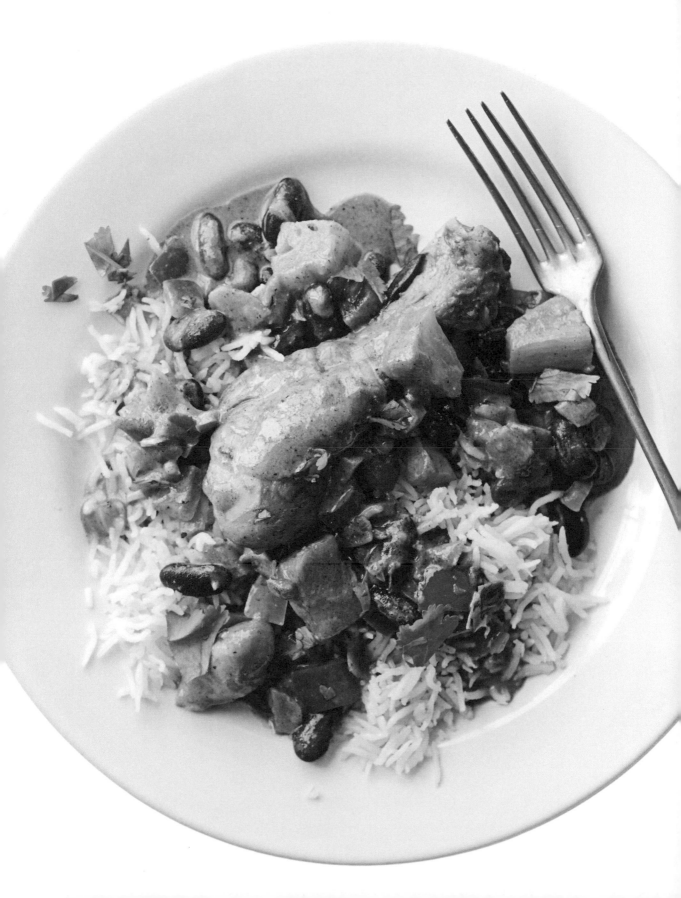

Stir-Fried Chicken with Broccoli & Brown Rice

Lean chicken and superhealthy broccoli make a great combo in stir-fries. Here chilli and fresh ginger with cholesterol-busting garlic pack in the flavours to go with them.

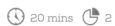 20 mins 2

- 200g/7oz trimmed broccoli florets, halved
- 1 large skinless chicken breast, diced
- 1 tsp mild chilli powder, or chipotle paste
- 2 tsp rapeseed oil
- 15g/½oz fresh ginger, shredded
- 2 garlic cloves, shredded
- 1 red onion, sliced
- 1 tbsp soy sauce, preferably reduced salt
- 1 tbsp clear honey
- 1 roasted red pepper from a jar, cubed
- 250g pack cooked brown basmati rice

1 Put the kettle on to boil and tip the broccoli in a medium pan ready to go on the heat. Mix the chicken with the chilli powder. Pour the water over the broccoli then boil for 4 mins.

2 Heat the oil in a non-stick wok and stir fry the ginger, garlic and onion for 2 mins. Add the chicken and stir-fry for 2 mins more. Drain the broccoli and reserve the water. Add the broccoli to the wok with the soy, honey, red pepper and 4 tbsp broccoli water then cook until heated through. Meanwhile, heat the pack of rice according to the instructions and serve with the stir-fry.

PER SERVING 448 kcals, fat 9g, saturates 2g, carbs 56g, sugars 15g, fibre 6g, protein 33g, salt 1.4g

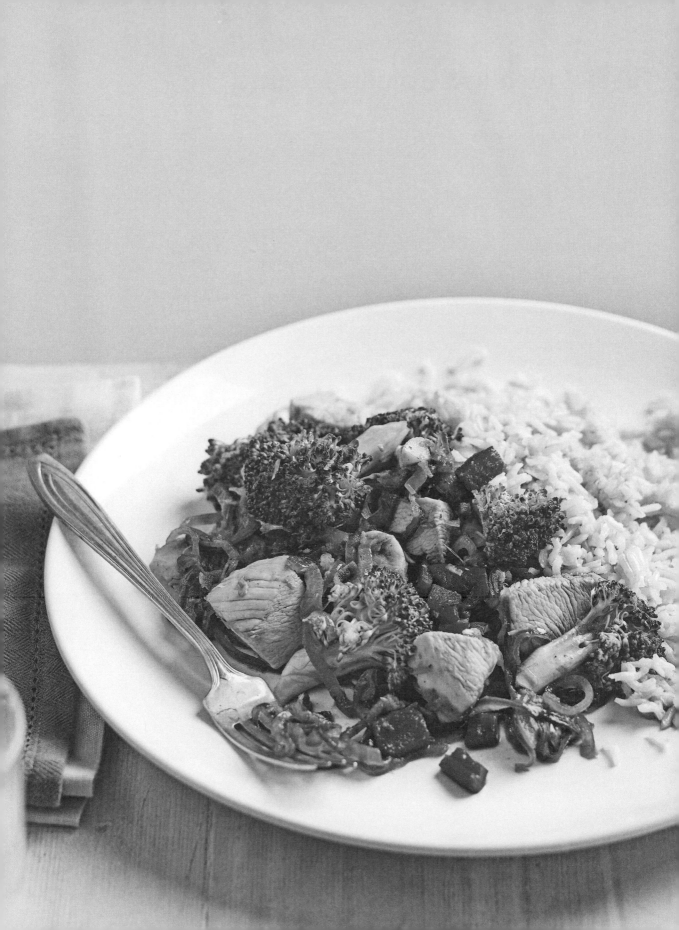

Asian Pulled Chicken Salad

You can rustle this up in next to no time with a bought cooked chicken. If you are halving the quantity to serve two you might even have leftover from a roast that you could use.

🕐 20 mins ◔ 4-5

- 1 small roasted chicken, about 1kg/2lb 4oz
- ½ red cabbage, cored and finely sliced
- 3 carrots, coarsely grated or finely shredded
- 5 spring onions, finely sliced on the diagonal
- 2 red chillies, halved and thinly sliced
- small bunch coriander, roughly chopped, including stalks
- 2 heaped tbsp roasted peanuts, roughly crushed

FOR THE DRESSING
- 3½ tbsp hoisin sauce
- 1½ tbsp sesame oil

1 Combine the dressing ingredients in a small bowl and set aside.
2 Remove all the meat from the chicken, shred into large chunks and pop in a large bowl. Add the cabbage, carrots, spring onions, chillies and half the coriander. Toss together with the dressing and pile onto a serving plate, then scatter over the remaining coriander and peanuts.

PER SERVING 352 kcals, fat 19g, saturates 4g, carbs 14g, sugars 11g, fibre 5g, protein 29g, salt 0.8g

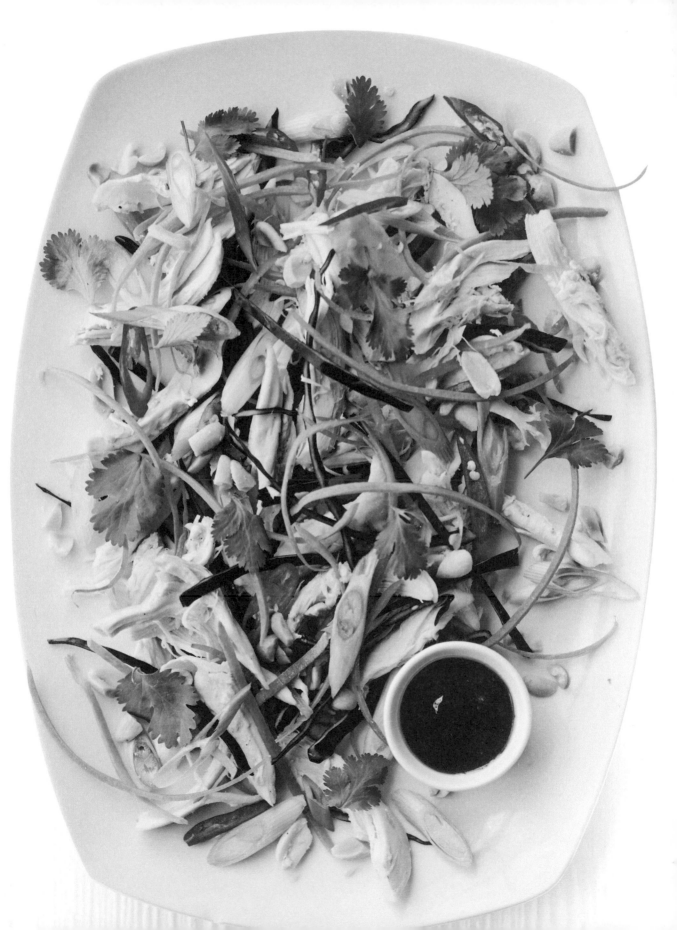

Chicken & Avocado Salad with Blueberry Dressing

Use leftover roast chicken or poach or pan-fry a chicken breast for this salad. Balsamic vinegar is worth having in your store cupboard; it really adds flavour to salad dressings.

🕐 20 mins 🥧 2

- 85g/3oz blueberries
- 1 tbsp rapeseed oil
- 2 tsp balsamic vinegar
- 125g/5½oz frozen baby broad beans or frozen soya beans
- 1 garlic clove, finely chopped
- 1 large cooked beetroot, finely chopped
- 1 avocado, halved, stoned, peeled and sliced
- 85g bag mixed baby leaf salad
- 175g/6oz cooked chicken, chopped

1 Mash half the blueberries with the oil, vinegar and some black pepper in a large salad bowl.
2 Boil the broad beans for 5 mins until just tender. Drain, leaving them unskinned.
3 Stir the garlic into the dressing, then pile in the warm beans and remaining blueberries with the beetroot, avocado, salad and chicken. Toss to mix, but don't go overboard or the juice from the beetroot will turn everything pink. Pile onto plates or into shallow bowls to serve.

PER SERVING 402 kcals, fat 19g, saturates 3g, carbs 18g, sugars 10g, fibre 10g, protein 34g, salt 0.3g

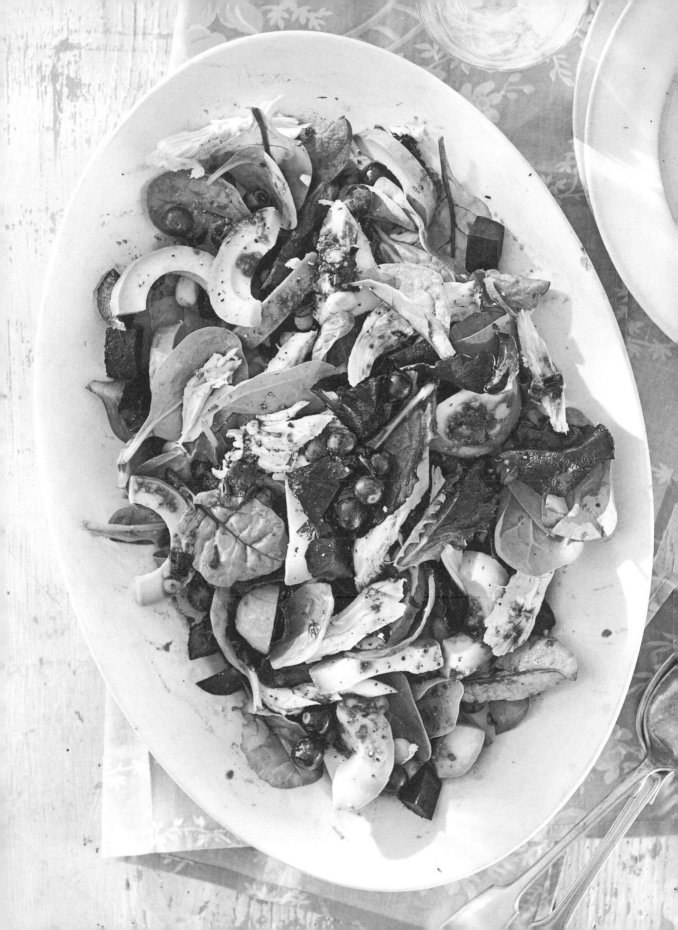

Griddled Chicken with Jade Mash

High-protein frozen soya beans, found in the freezer section along with peas, makes the mash for this.

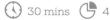 30 mins 4

- 2 garlic cloves, crushed
- zest and juice 1½ lemons
- 2 tbsp toasted sesame oil
- 4 small skinless chicken breasts, cut in half lengthways to make 8 flat pieces
- 300g/11oz frozen soya beans
- 500g/1lb 2oz frozen peas
- 1 red onion, finely chopped
- 1–2 red chillies, deseeded and chopped
- thumb-sized piece ginger, peeled and finely grated
- 100g/4oz low-fat natural yogurt

1 Mix the garlic, two-thirds of the lemon zest and juice, and 1 tbsp sesame oil in a large bowl. Add the chicken and mix to coat.

2 Put a large saucepan of water on to boil. Tip in the beans, boil for 4 mins, then add the peas and cook for another 2 mins. Drain and set aside.

3 Return the pan to the heat with the remaining sesame oil, the onion, chilli and ginger, and cook for 4 mins until just beginning to soften. Tip the beans and peas back into the pan and roughly crush with a potato masher. Turn off the heat and stir in the yogurt and remaining lemon zest and juice. Add a splash of water if you need to.

4 Meanwhile, heat a griddle pan over a medium-high heat and cook the chicken for 3–4 mins each side until charred and cooked through. Divide the mash between four plates, top with the griddled chicken and serve.

PER SERVING 428 kcals, fat 14g, saturates 3g, carbs 22g, sugars 7g, fibre 13g, protein 46g, salt 0.2g

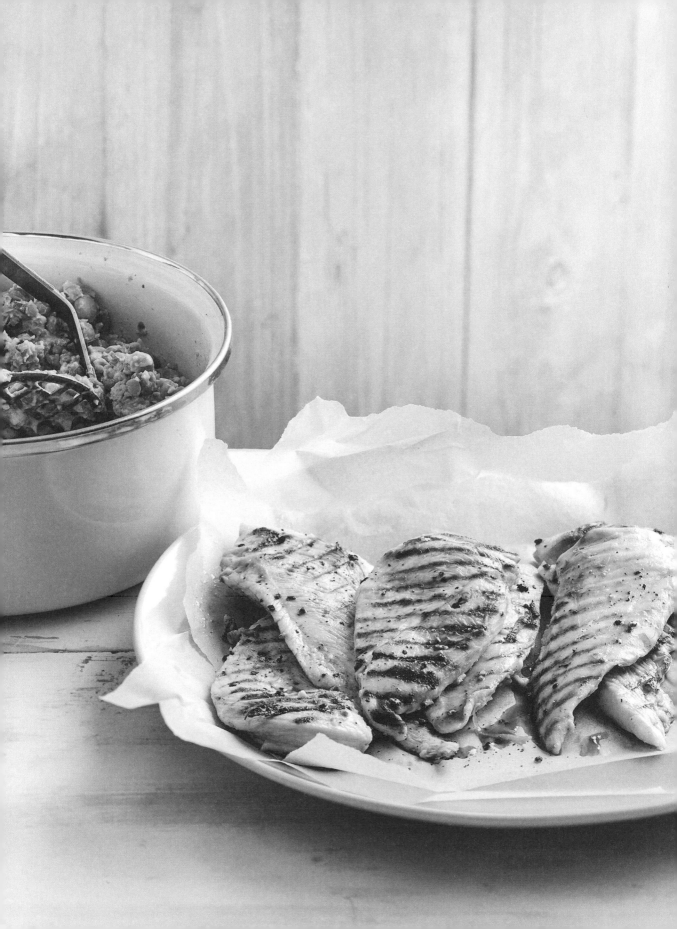

Chipotle Chicken with Corn & Pepper Pilaf

Fresh corn makes an interesting and really delicious alternative to rice in this pilaf, a perfect late-summer recipe when corn is cheap and in season.

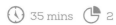 35 mins 2

- 1 lime, zest and juice of ½, the other ½ cut into wedges
- 1 tbsp chipotle paste or 1 tsp smoked paprika
- 1 tbsp rapeseed oil
- 2 skinless chicken breast fillets
- 1 large onion, finely chopped
- 1 red pepper, deseeded and finely diced
- 1 tsp cumin seeds
- 1 red chilli, deseeded and finely chopped
- 2 corn cobs
- small pack coriander, a few leaves reserved, the rest chopped

1 Mix the lime zest and juice with the chipotle paste and 2 tsp oil in a bowl. Cut each chicken breast into diagonal slices to make 3–4 fillets, add to the bowl and toss until well coated.

2 Heat the remaining oil in a non-stick pan, add the onion and fry for 10 mins, stirring frequently, until softened. Add the pepper, cumin seeds and chilli and cook for 5 mins more. Meanwhile, slice down the sides of the corn cobs with a sharp knife to remove the kernels.

3 Heat a large non-stick frying pan, add the chicken and cook for 5 mins, turning once, until cooked through but still juicy. Add the corn to the pepper mixture and cook for 3–4 mins. Stir in the chopped coriander and serve with the chicken, with coriander leaves sprinkled over and the lime wedges on the side.

PER SERVING 438 kcals, fat 11g, saturates 1g, carbs 42g, sugars 16g, fibre 9g, protein 39g, salt 0.4g

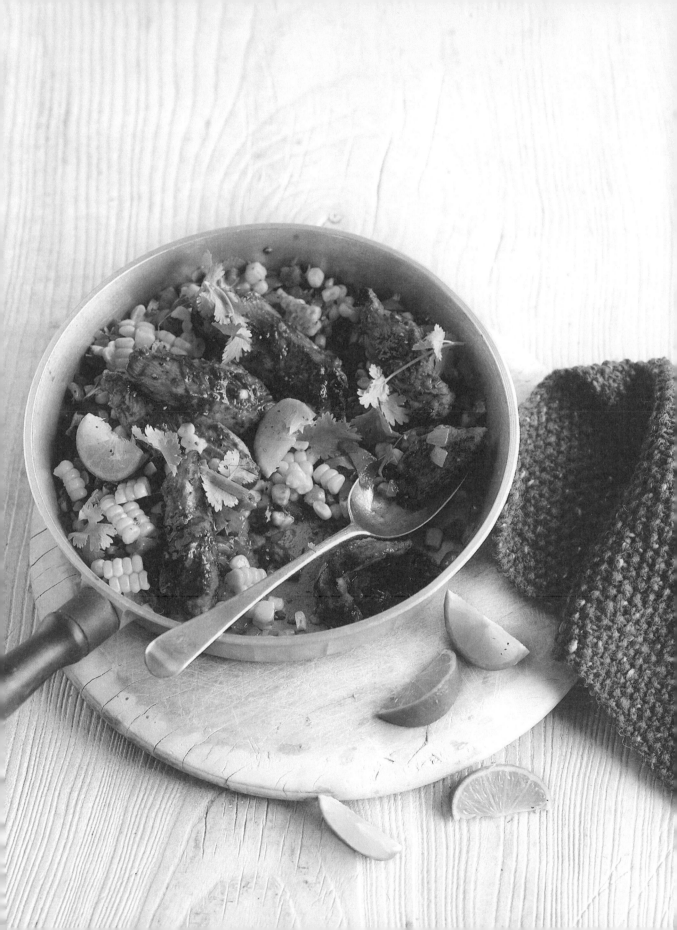

Chicken Schnitzel with Coleslaw

Children will recognise this as a posh version of chicken nuggets, but they are served with a healthy coleslaw, using yogurt as the dressing instead of mayo.

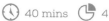 40 mins 4

FOR THE SCHNITZEL
- 4 small skinless chicken breasts
- 100g/4oz plain flour
- 1 large egg, beaten
- 75g/2½oz dried breadcrumbs
- 3 tbsp grated Parmesan
- 75ml/2½fl oz rapeseed oil

FOR THE COLESLAW
- 300g/11oz white cabbage, shredded
- 1 large carrot, peeled and grated
- 6 spring onions, sliced diagonally
- 1 red-skinned apple, grated
- 150g pot natural yogurt
- juice ½ lemon
- 2 tsp English mustard

1 For the coleslaw, mix all the ingredients in a large bowl and set aside.

2 Place a layer of cling film on your work surface and put the chicken breast fillets on top. Cover with another piece of cling film and, using a rolling pin, bash the chicken until it is 2–3mm thick.

3 Put the flour on a plate, then put the egg on another plate. Dip the chicken in the flour to coat, then into the egg.

4 Mix together the breadcrumbs and Parmesan in a shallow bowl, then toss the chicken in the mixture to completely coat in the crumbs. Put the chicken on a plate and chill in the fridge until ready to eat if you're not cooking them straight away.

5 Heat the oil in a large frying pan over a fairly high heat and cook the chicken schnitzels two at a time. Sizzle them for 2–3 mins each side until completely golden, then lift out onto kitchen paper to drain. You can keep them warm in a low oven while you cook the rest. Serve with the coleslaw.

PER SERVING 430 kcals, fat 19g, saturates 5g, carbs 26g, sugars 13g, fibre 5g, protein 36g, salt 1.1g

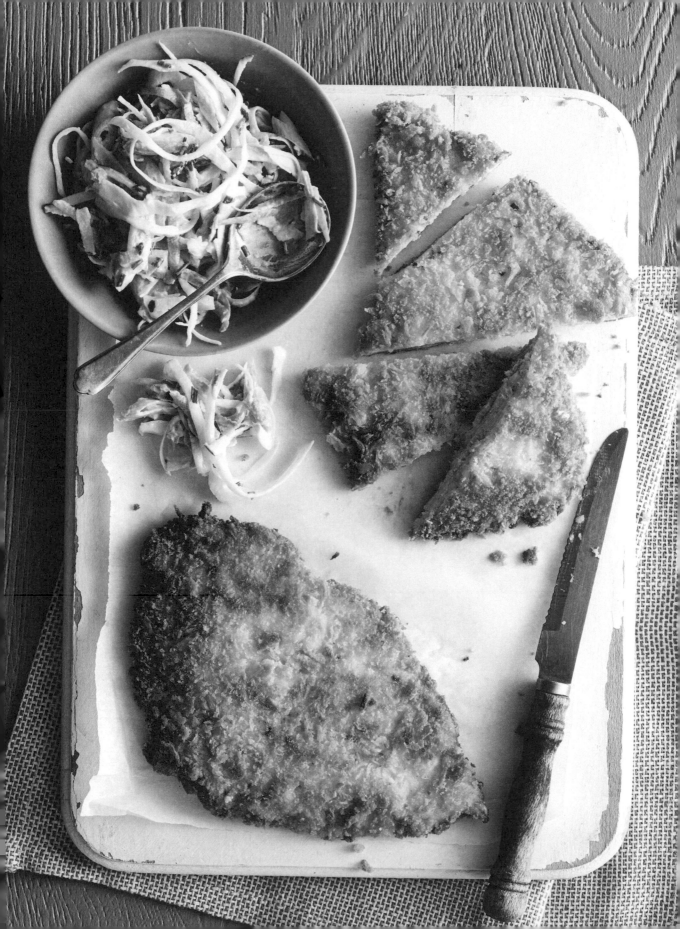

Spinach, Ricotta & Chicken Traybake

Low in fat, high in fibre, 4 of your 5 a day and tasty enough for entertaining friends – what could be better?

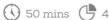 50 mins 4

- 3 x 100g bags baby spinach
- 4 tbsp ricotta
- zest and juice 1 lemon
- a few grinds of nutmeg
- 4 skinless chicken breasts
- 2 tbsp olive oil
- 50g/2oz fresh breadcrumbs
- 3 courgettes, cut into batons
- 2 peppers, deseeded and sliced
- 2 red onions, cut into wedges, roots intact
- 250g/9oz vine cherry tomatoes
- 4 garlic cloves

1 Heat oven to 200C/180C fan/gas 6. Put the spinach in a large colander and pour over 1–2 kettles of boiling water to wilt it. Allow to drain for a few mins, then squeeze out as much excess water as possible. Chop, put in a bowl and beat in the ricotta, lemon zest, nutmeg and plenty of black pepper.

2 Using a sharp knife, cut a slit into the side of each chicken breast and use your fingers to make a little pocket. Spoon the mixture into the 4 breasts. Rub with 2 tsp of the oil and press the breadcrumbs on top, then arrange the chicken in a roasting tin.

3 Put the vegetables on another tray and drizzle with the remaining oil, and season well. Bake the chicken and veg for around 30 mins, stirring the veg once. Remove when the chicken is cooked through and the breadcrumbs are golden.

4 Remove the softened garlic from the vegetables and mash it with the lemon juice, then stir this with the roasted veg and serve with the chicken.

PER SERVING 348 kcals, fat 11g, saturates 3g, carbs 24g, sugars 9g, fibre 6g, protein 39g, salt 0.8g

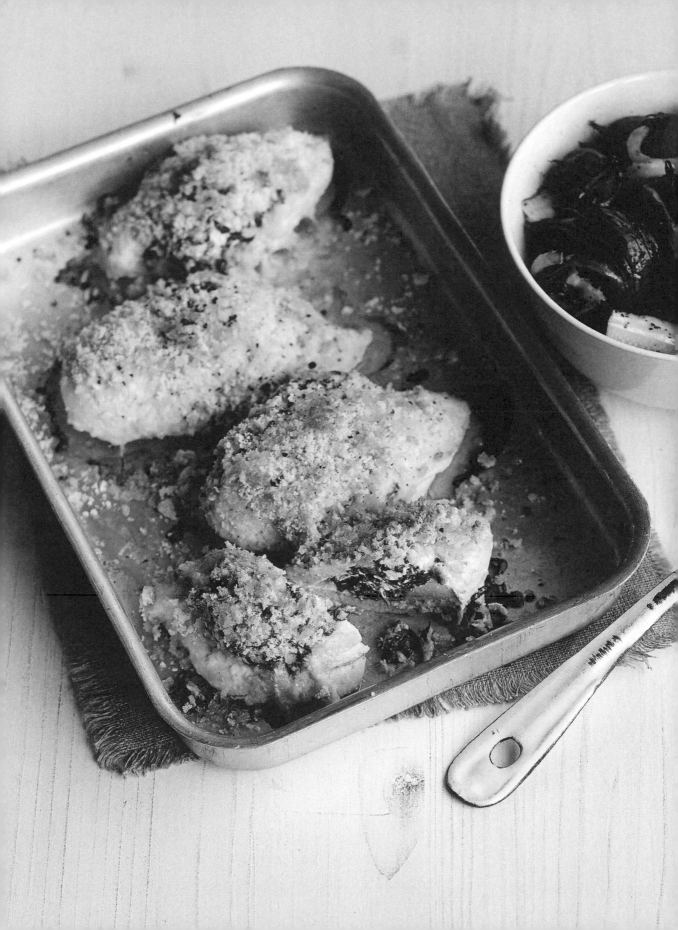

Turkey Enchiladas

Turkey mince is substantially lower in fat than beef mince and is well worth using in family dishes like these tasty Mexican tortillas baked with cheese.

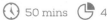 50 mins 4

- 1 tbsp rapeseed oil
- 500g/1lb 2oz turkey mince (2% fat)
- 1 medium onion, finely chopped
- 1 yellow pepper, deseeded and thinly sliced
- 400g can chopped tomatoes
- 400g can red kidney beans in chilli sauce
- 1 tbsp fresh lime or lemon juice
- 2 heaped tbsp roughly chopped coriander, plus extra to garnish
- 6 regular or 8 mini flour tortillas
- 50g/2oz reduced-fat mature Cheddar, coarsely grated
- large mixed salad, to serve

1 Heat oven to 200C/180C fan/gas 6. Heat most of the oil in a large non-stick frying pan. Fry the turkey, onion and pepper for 5 mins, stirring regularly and breaking up the mince with a wooden spoon. Add the chopped tomatoes and kidney beans.

2 Bring to a gentle simmer and cook for 10 mins, stirring regularly. Remove from the heat and stir in the lime or lemon juice and coriander.

3 Lightly grease a shallow ovenproof dish with the remaining oil. Put 1 tortilla in the dish and top with a couple of generous spoonfuls of the turkey mixture. Roll up and push to one side of the dish. Repeat with the other tortillas, then spoon any remaining turkey mixture down the sides of the dish.

4 Sprinkle the tortillas with the cheese and bake for 15 mins. Scatter coriander over the enchiladas and serve with a mixed salad.

PER SERVING 486 kcals, fat 8g, saturates 3g, carbs 56g, sugars 12g, fibre 9g, protein 44g, salt 1.6g

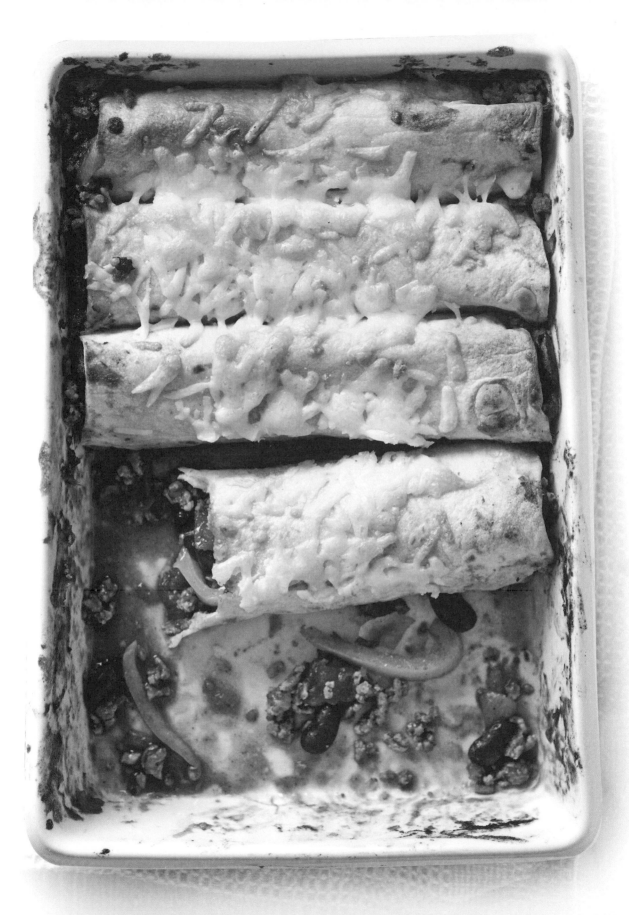

Spicy Turkey Sweet Potatoes

These are low fat, even with a soured cream topping, the secret is the turkey mince. The filling would be delicious with normal baked potatoes, but sweet ones offer better nutrition.

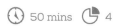 50 mins 4

- 4 sweet potatoes
- 1 tbsp rapeseed oil
- 1 onion, finely chopped
- 1 garlic clove, crushed
- 500g pack turkey thigh mince
- 500g carton passata
- 3 tbsp barbecue or hoisin sauce
- ½ tsp smoked paprika
- 4 tbsp soured cream or yogurt
- ½ pack chives, finely snipped

1 Heat oven to 200C/180C fan/gas 6. Prick the potatoes, place on a baking tray and bake for 45 mins or until really soft.

2 Meanwhile, heat the oil in a frying pan, add the onion and cook gently for 8 mins until softened. Stir in the garlic, then tip in the mince and stir to break up. Cook over a high heat until any liquid has evaporated and the mince is browned, about 10 mins. Pour in the passata, then fill the carton a quarter full of water and tip that in, too. Add the barbecue sauce and paprika, then lower the heat and simmer gently for 15 mins, adding a little extra water if needed.

3 When the potatoes are soft, split them down the centre and spoon the mince over the top. Add a dollop of soured cream or yogurt and a sprinkling of chives.

PER SERVING 464 kcals, fat 10g, saturates 4g, carbs 58g, sugars 35g, fibre 10g, protein 31g, salt 0.9g

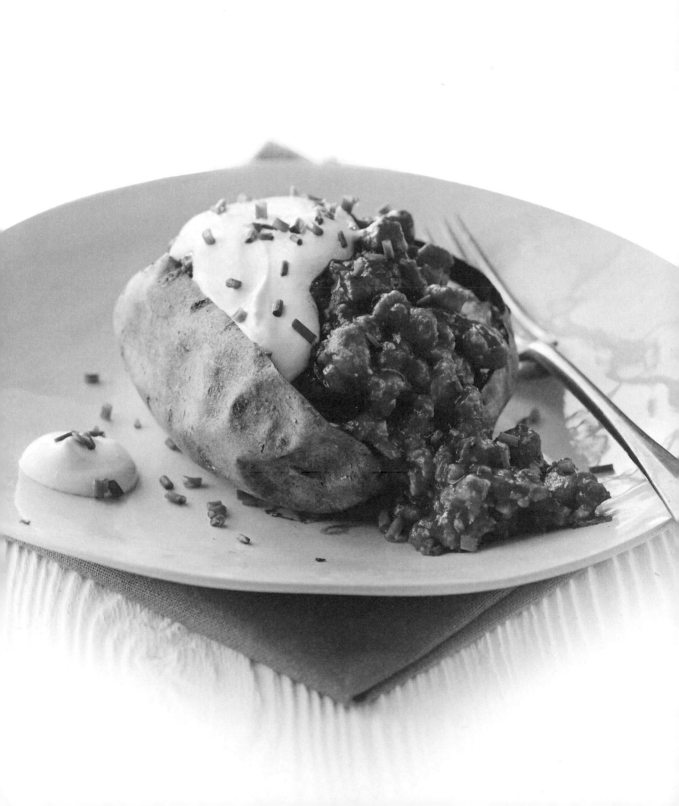

Chipolatas in Apple Gravy with Parsnip Colcannon

Try not to eat too many products like sausage, but when you do, choose ones with a high meat content.

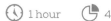 1 hour 4

- 1 large potato, cut into chunks
- 4 parsnips, peeled and cut into chunks
- 8 low-fat chipolatas
- 25g/1oz butter
- 2 large red apples, cored and cut into slim wedges
- 8 spring onions, sliced, white and green parts separated
- 200g/7oz kale or Savoy cabbage, finely chopped
- 1 tbsp plain flour
- 1 beef or chicken stock cube
- 50ml/2fl oz skimmed milk

1 Put the potato and parsnips in a very large pan of water, bring to the boil and simmer for 10 mins or until the veg is tender.

2 Meanwhile, cook the chipolatas in a large frying pan. When brown on all sides, transfer to a plate and add half the butter to the pan. Add the apples and white part of the spring onions. Fry for 5–10 mins until softened and starting to caramelise.

3 Add the kale to the boiling veg for the final few mins, before the potatoes and parsnips are completely soft. When the kale has wilted, drain the veg and leave to steam-dry in the colander. Heat the remaining butter in the same pan – don't worry about washing it out. Add the green parts of the spring onions and sizzle for a few mins to soften.

4 Add the flour and stock cube to the apples and spring onions, stir for 1–2 mins, then add 400ml water, mixing to a smooth gravy. Return the sausages to the pan and bubble in the gravy for a few mins until heated through.

5 Meanwhile, add the veg to the spring onions, along with the milk, and mash until the potato and parsnips are smooth. Serve the colcannon with the chipolatas and the gravy spooned over the top.

PER SERVING 419 kcals, fat 11g, saturates 5g, carbs 57g, sugars 24g, fibre 12g, protein 15g, salt 1.6g

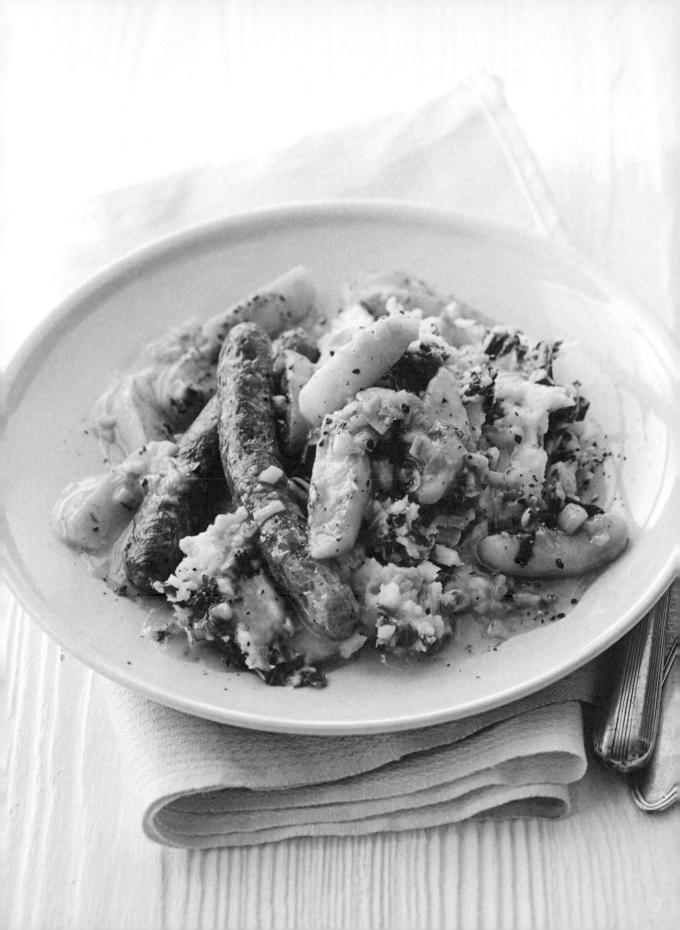

Pork & Parsnip Traybake

Serve this with green veg like stir-fried cabbage or broccoli or a few rocket leaves.

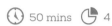 50 mins 4

- 4 large parsnips (about 500g/1lb 3oz), peeled and cut lengthways into 6
- 2 red onions, each cut into 8 wedges through the root
- 2½ tbsp olive oil
- 1½ tbsp wholegrain mustard
- 4 pork chops, fat trimmed
- 1½ tbsp clear honey
- small handful sage leaves

1 Heat oven to 220C/200C fan/gas 7. Put the vegetables in a roasting tin, season and toss with 2 tbsp oil and 1 tbsp mustard.
2 Roast for 20 mins. Meanwhile, place a frying pan over a high heat. Season the pork chops and rub with the remaining oil. Fry the chops for 30 secs–1 min each side until just browned – turn on their sides to brown any fat.
3 Stir the veg, then place the chops on top and rub them with the remaining mustard the roast for a further 15 mins. Drizzle with honey and scatter over the sage, then return to the oven for 5 mins or until the pork is cooked through. Serve with the juices from the tin.

PER SERVING 574 kcals, fat 29g, saturates 5g, carbs 26g, sugars 16g, fibre 9g, protein 47g, salt 0.7g

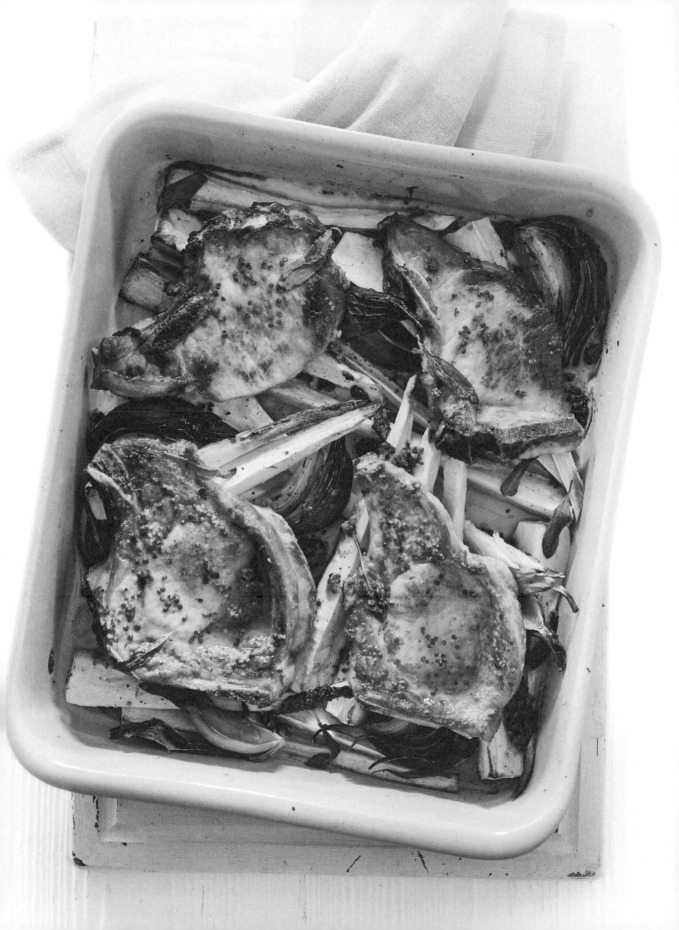

Pork, Lime & Cashew Stir-fry

This stir-fry is fresh and zingy with beansprouts and cabbage as well as the crunch of cashews. If you want a bit of heat add a little Thai red curry paste, or sweet chilli sauce.

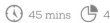 45 mins 4

- 600g/1lb 5oz pork loin steaks, trimmed and cut into thin strips
- 2 tbsp soy sauce, preferably reduced-salt
- 2 limes, zest and juice of 1½, ½ cut into wedges, to serve
- 300g/11oz basmati rice or brown rice
- 1–2 tbsp rapeseed oil, for frying
- 2 bunches spring onions, trimmed and cut into thirds
- 300g bag beansprouts
- 1 Savoy or sweetheart cabbage (about 300g/11oz), shredded
- 25g/1oz cashews, roughly chopped

1 Tip the pork into a medium bowl. Stir together the soy sauce, lime zest and juice, pour over the pork and mix well, then set aside.

2 Put a medium pan of water on to boil. Tip in the rice and cook following the pack instructions. Meanwhile, heat 1 tbsp oil in a large non-stick frying pan or wok over a high heat and add the spring onions. Cook for 1–2 mins until golden brown and softened. Lift out of the pan onto a plate lined with kitchen paper.

3 Return the frying pan to the heat. If the pan is dry, add another 1 tbsp oil. Tip in the pork and marinade, and stir-fry over a high heat for 4–5 mins until the pork is nearly cooked. Tip in the beansprouts and cabbage, and stir-fry for another 3 mins until the pork is cooked through and the vegetables are slightly soft. Stir in the spring onions, sprinkle over the cashews and serve with the rice and lime wedges.

PER SERVING 569 kcals, fat 13g, saturates 2g, carbs 66g, sugars 5g, fibre 5g, protein 45g, salt 0.9g

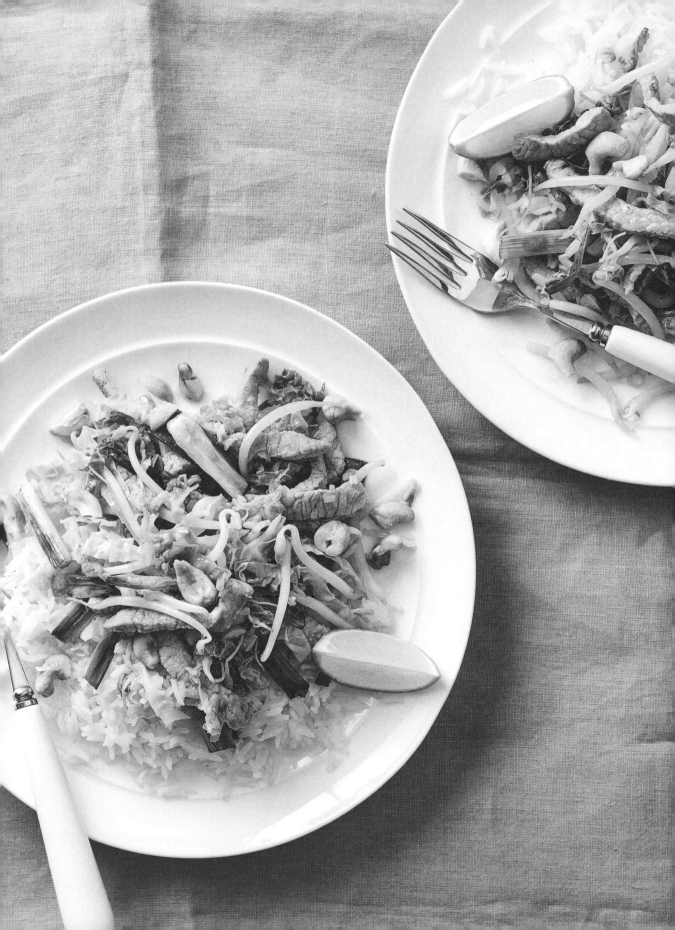

Home-style Pork Curry with Cauliflower Rice

Who would imagine that a curry could be low-fat, low-calorie and packed with vitamin C, let alone provide 4 of your 5 a day!

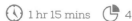 1 hr 15 mins 4

FOR THE CURRY
- 425g/15oz lean pork fillet (tenderloin), cubed
- 2 tbsp Madras curry paste or powder
- 2 tbsp red or white wine vinegar
- 1 tbsp rapeseed oil
- 1 large onion, finely chopped
- 2 tbsp finely shredded ginger
- 1 tsp each fennel and cumin seeds, toasted in a pan then crushed
- 400g can chopped tomatoes
- 2 tbsp red lentils
- 350g pack baby aubergine, quartered or 1 large aubergine, cut into cubes
- 1 vegetable or chicken stock cube

FOR THE CAULIFLOWER RICE
- 1 medium cauliflower
- good handful chopped coriander

1 Tip the pork into a bowl and stir in the curry paste or powder and vinegar. Set aside. Heat the oil in a heavy based pan and fry the onion and ginger for 10 mins, stirring frequently until golden. Tip in the pork mixture and fry a few mins more. Remove the pork and put to one side. Stir in the toasted spices then tip in the tomatoes, the lentils and aubergine then crumble in the stock cube. Cover and leave to simmer for 40 mins, stirring frequently, until the aubergine is nearly cooked. If it starts to look dry, add a splash of water. Return the pork to the pan and cook for a further 10–20 mins until the pork is cooked and tender.

2 Just before serving, cut the hard core and stalks from the cauliflower and pulse in a food processor to make grains the size of rice. Tip into a Pyrex bowl, cover with cling film then pierce and cook for 7 mins on High. There is no need to add any water. Stir through the coriander and serve with the curry. For spicy rice, add some toasted cumin seeds.

PER SERVING 309 kcals, fat 10g, saturates 2g, carbs 18g, sugars 11g, fibre 9g, protein 33g, salt 0.6g

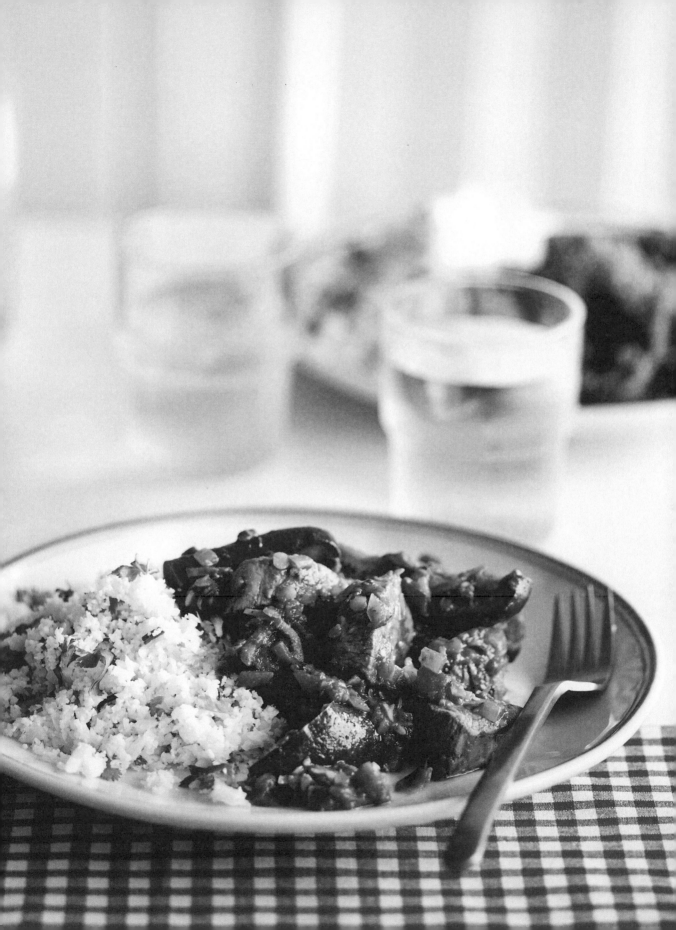

Pork with Orange & Rosemary

This is served with a tasty pea and broccoli crush, a bit like mash, but new potatoes cooked in their skins will go well with this, too.

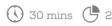 30 mins 2

- 1 tsp rapeseed oil
- 5 shallots, halved
- 2 x 100g/4oz pieces lean pork fillet, all visible fat removed
- 2 sprigs rosemary
- 150ml/¼ pint chicken stock
- 1 tsp smoked paprika
- 1 tsp clear honey
- 1 orange

FOR THE BROCOLI & PEA CRUSH

- 200g/7oz broccoli, cut into small florets
- 3 spring onions, chopped
- 100g/4oz frozen petits pois

1 Heat the oil in a non-stick frying pan, add the shallots cut side down, then cover and cook for 8–10 mins, until the shallots have softened. Add the pork and rosemary to the pan and fry, turning the meat to seal it.

2 Pour in the stock, stir in the paprika and honey, then cover the pan and cook gently for 10 mins.

3 Meanwhile, boil the broccoli and spring onions in a covered pan for 5 mins then add the petits pois and cook 5 mins more until tender. Drain, then crush with a masher.

4 Cut the peel and pith from the orange with a sharp knife, then cut between the membrane to make segments. Add any juice to the pork. When the pork is cooked, remove from the heat and toss through the segments. Serve with the vegetable crush.

PER SERVING 276 kcals, fat 7g, saturates 1g, carbs 16g, sugars 12g, fibre 9g, protein 32g, salt 0.4g

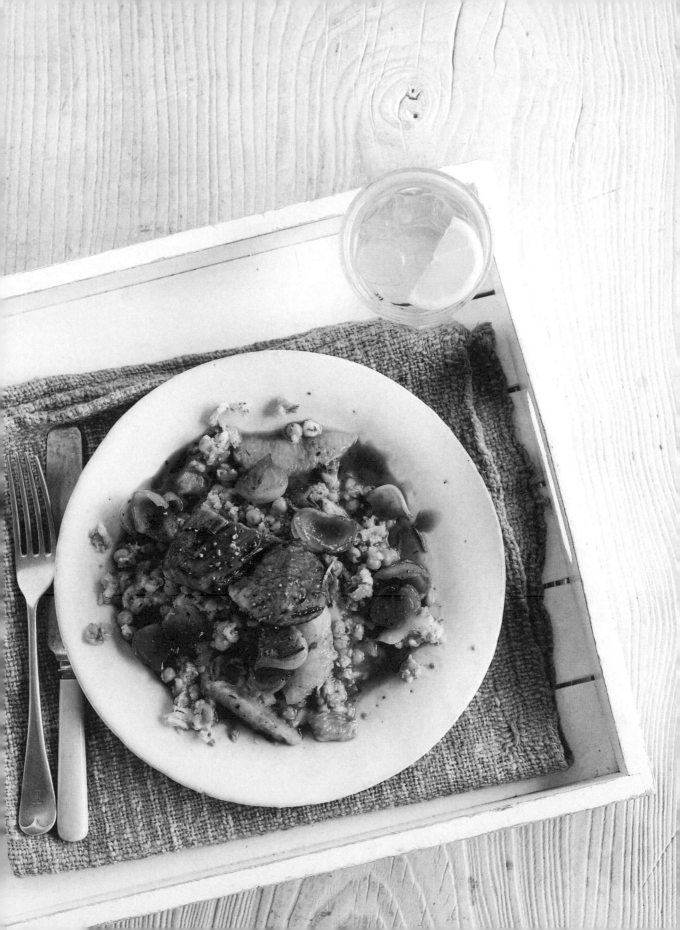

Pulled Ham & Maple Mustard Slaw

Take out the ham and this slaw will make a great side to serve with slices of leftover meat from a Sunday roast.

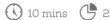 10 mins 2

- 2 tsp rapeseed oil
- 1 tbsp white wine vinegar
- ¼ tsp grainy mustard
- 2 tsp maple syrup or clear honey
- ⅓ small red cabbage, shredded
- 6 ready to eat dried apricots, cut into strips
- 1 red onion, finely chopped
- 6 walnut halves, broken into pieces
- 2–3 tbsp chopped parsley
- 100g/4oz piece of ham, pulled into pieces

1 Mix the oil, vinegar, mustard and maple syrup in a bowl then stir in the cabbage, apricots, onion, walnuts and parsley and toss well. Now gently fold through the ham.

PER SERVING 260 kcals, fat 12g, saturates 2g, carbs 22g, sugars 20g, fibre 7g, protein 14g, salt 1.7g

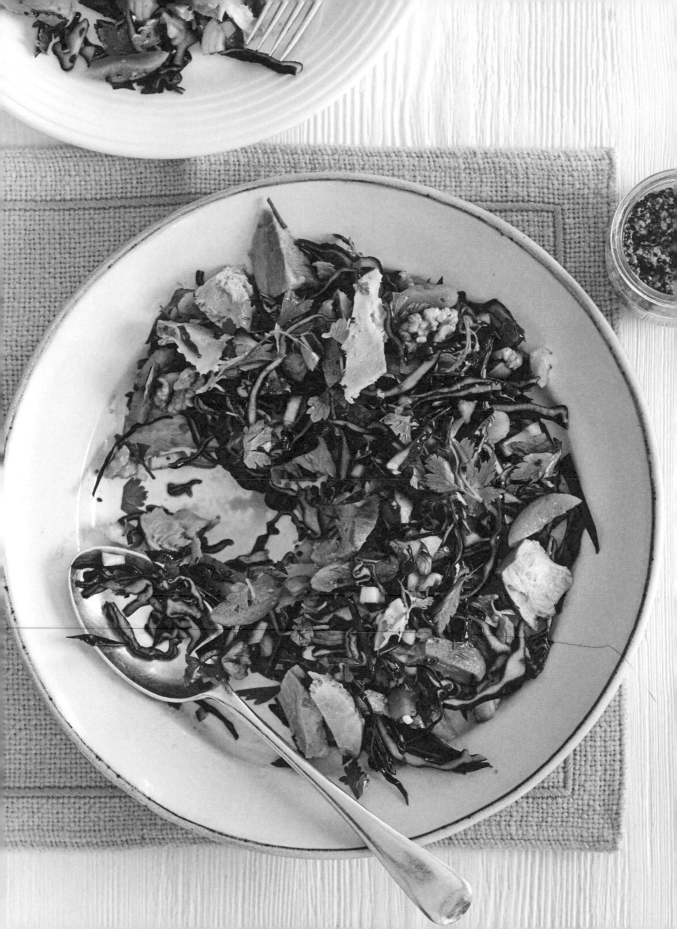

Pearl Barley, Bacon & Leek Casserole

Barley is a cheap and underused store-cupboard grain that makes a great alternative to rice. It is teamed here with bacon and veggies for a risotto-like stew, rich in fibre and iron.

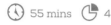 55 mins | 4

- 1 tbsp olive or rapeseed oil
- 2 leeks, thickly sliced
- 2 garlic cloves, finely chopped
- 300g/11oz pearl barley
- 4 carrots, cubed
- 1 tbsp Dijon or wholegrain mustard, plus extra to serve
- 1 litre/1¾ pints chicken stock
- 300g/11oz Savoy cabbage, shredded
- 200g/7oz back bacon, chopped into small pieces

1 Heat a large pan over a medium heat. Add the oil and cook the leeks for a few mins, then add the garlic and cook for just 1 min more.

2 Add the pearl barley, carrots and mustard, then pour over the chicken stock. Season with plenty of ground black pepper and simmer for 20 mins, stirring occasionally. Add the cabbage with the bacon, and cook for 5–10 mins until the cabbage is wilted and tender. Serve with extra mustard on the side.

PER SERVING 589 kcals, fat 15g, saturates 3g, carbs 73g, sugars 11g, fibre 8g, protein 43g, salt 0.8g

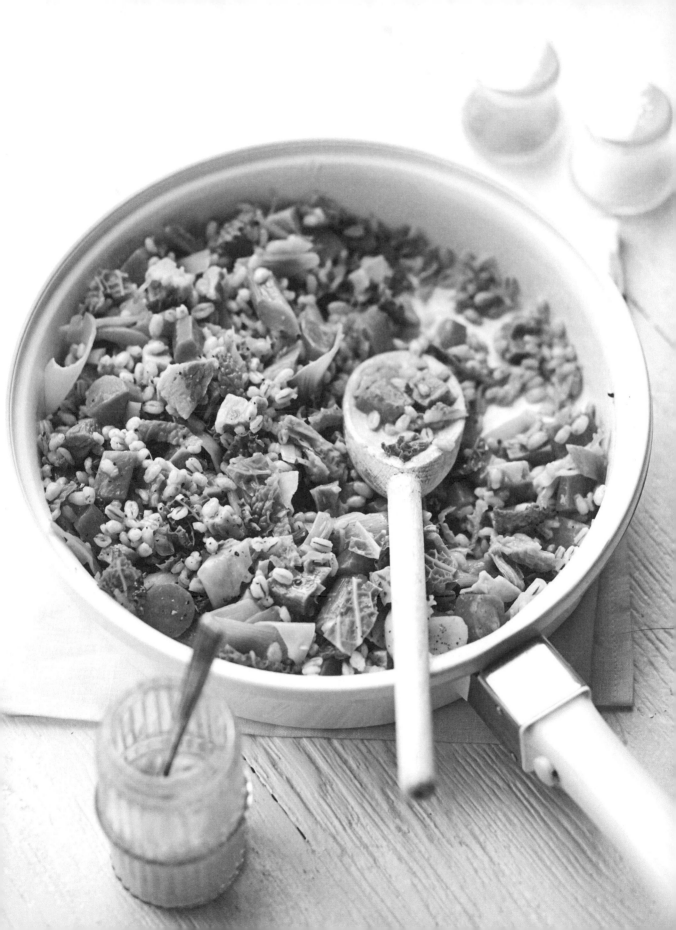

Greek Lamb with Smoked Aubergine & Minty Broad Beans

Many people assume that red meat is bad for you, but eaten in moderation it offers protein, iron and valuable B vitamins. This makes a good choice for a bbq.

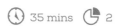 35 mins 2

- 1 aubergine
- ½ lemon, zest and juice, plus wedges to serve
- 2 large garlic cloves, finely grated
- 1 tsp fresh oregano or ½ tsp dried
- 2 tsp extra virgin olive oil, plus ½ tsp
- 2 lean leg lamb steaks, about 100g/4oz each, all visible fat removed
- 100g/4oz frozen baby broad beans or soya beans
- 2 tbsp Greek bio yogurt
- 2 tsp tahini
- 12 mint leaves, roughly torn

1 Turn on your largest gas flame and cook the aubergine on top of it, turning it every 2 mins for about 7–8 mins until it is soft and the skins have charred. You can do this on the bbq if you don't have a gas hob. Allow to cool a little.

2 Meanwhile, mix the lemon zest, half the garlic, oregano, some black pepper and ½ tsp oil then use this to coat the lamb steaks. Boil the beans for 4 mins.

3 Put the aubergine on a large plate and carefully remove and discard the skin, then finely chop the flesh, which should now be soft and pulpy, with a knife and fork. Tip into a bowl and stir with the remaining garlic, yogurt, seasoning and tahini and stir well.

4 Griddle or bbq the lamb for 5 mins, turning once. Meanwhile, mix the beans with the lemon juice, remaining olive oil and mint leaves. Spoon the aubergine purée onto plates and scatter round the minty beans. Top with the lamb and lemon wedges then serve.

PER SERVING 366 kcals, fat 19g, saturates 7g, carbs 13g, sugars 7g, fibre 11g, protein 30g, salt 0.2g

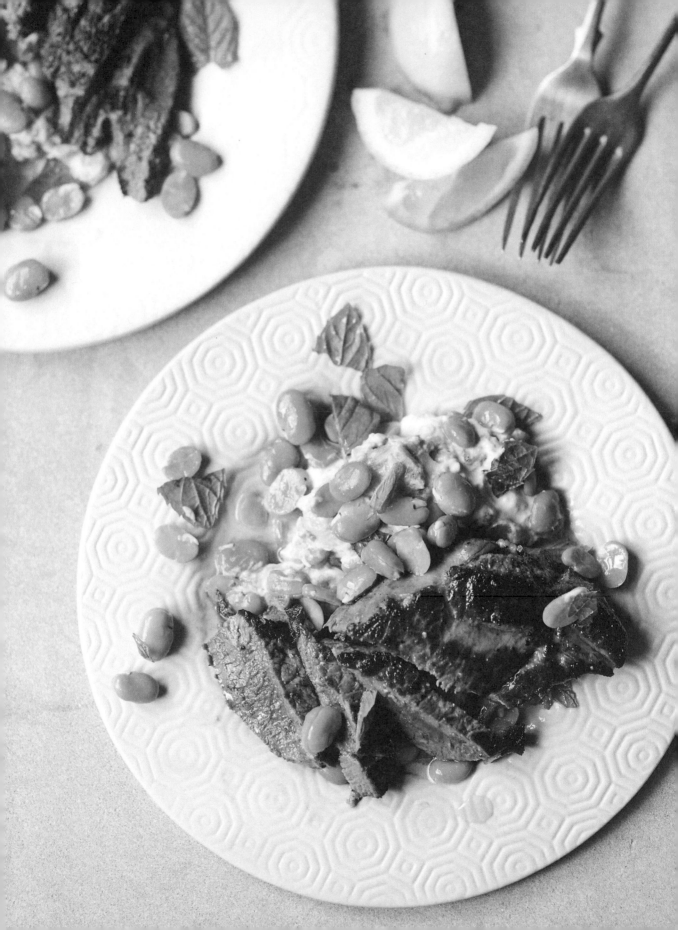

Bombay Lamb Wraps

Spice up cheap frozen lamb mince and vegetables and pile on wraps or chapatis for a healthy and filling dinner that teenagers will love.

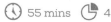 55 mins 4

- 1 tbsp rapeseed oil
- 1 large red onion, chopped
- 3 fat garlic cloves, crushed
- 200g/7oz frozen lamb mince
- 3 tbsp tikka masala or Madras curry paste
- 400g can chopped tomatoes
- 2 large potatoes, cut into cubes
- 250g/9oz frozen peas
- 8 flour wraps or chapatis, warmed
- 140g/5oz natural yogurt

1 Heat the oil in a large pan, add the onion and cook for a few mins to soften. Add the garlic, stir for 1 min, then add the frozen mince. Cook until defrosted and nicely browned, then stir in the curry paste, tomatoes, potatoes and half a can of water. Season well, then cover with a lid and simmer for 20 mins or until the potatoes are nearly cooked.

2 Remove the lid and simmer for a further 10–15 mins until the liquid has reduced and the sauce clings to the potatoes and mince. Add the peas, stir through until defrosted, then serve with the warm wraps and yogurt.

PER SERVING 576 kcals, fat 15g, saturates 4g, carbs 80g, sugars 12g, fibre 11g, protein 26g, salt 1.3g

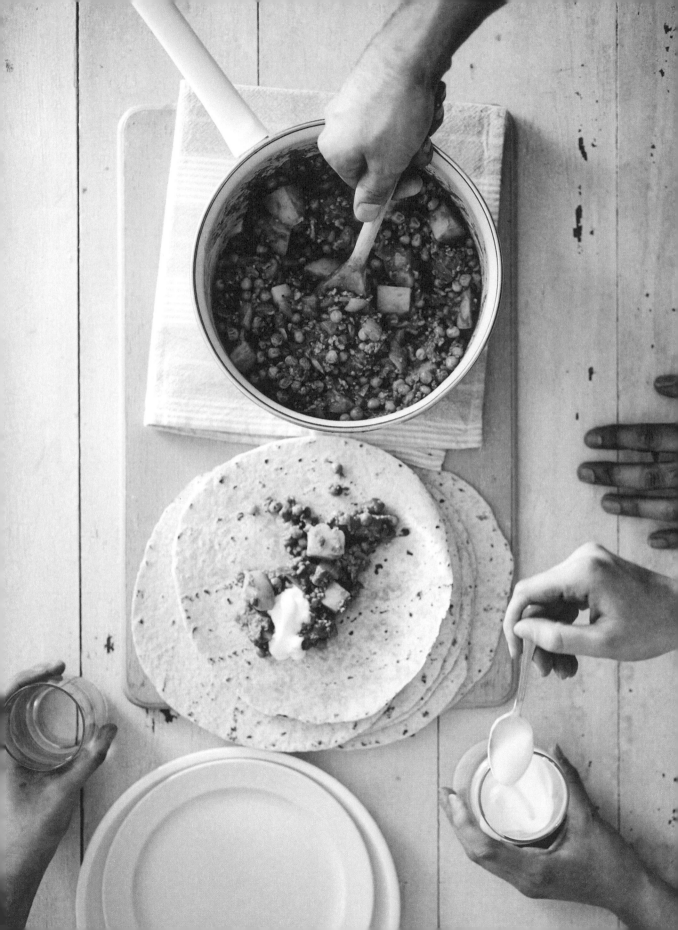

Chunky Chilli

This uses chunks of stewing beef instead of the usual mince for a more robust texture. Serve with rice or mash, or baked sweet potatoes and slaw.

🕐 2 hours 20 mins ◗ 4

- 1–2 tbsp rapeseed oil
- 400g/14oz lean diced stewing beef
- 1 onion, finely chopped
- 2 garlic cloves, finely chopped
- 1½ tsp ground cumin
- 1–2 tbsp chipotle paste depending on how spicy you like it or 1–2 tsp smoked paprika
- 400g can kidney beans in chilli sauce
- 400g can chopped tomatoes
- 1 lime, zested and cut into wedges
- ¼ small pack coriander, leaves only

1 Heat most of the oil in a large pan and cook the beef pieces for a few mins on each side until browned all over. Remove from the pan with a slotted spoon and set aside.

2 Add the onion to the pan, with extra oil if needed, and cook until softened. Stir in the garlic, cumin and chipotle paste and cook for 1 min. Drain the kidney beans, reserving the sauce. Add this sauce, along with the chopped tomatoes and a can full of water, to the pan. Stir well, then return the meat to the pan. Bring to a simmer, then cook, covered, for 2 hrs or until the beef is tender (or bake in the oven for 3 hrs at 160C/140C fan/gas 3).

3 Add the kidney beans and lime zest and warm through. Serve with a scattering of coriander leaves and the lime wedges to squeeze over.

PER SERVING 300 kcals, fat 13g, saturates 3g,carbs 21g, sugars 10g, fibre 6g, protein 26g, salt 0.9g

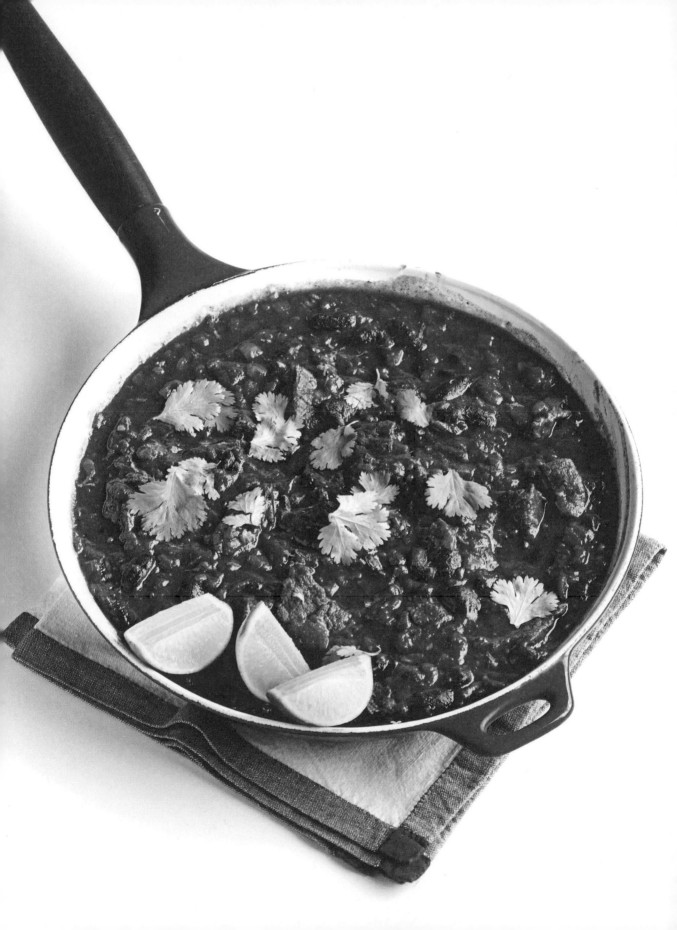

Lighter Beef Stew & Dumplings

Guilt-free comfort food at its very best. If you don't have wine you can just replace this with more stock.

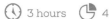 3 hours 4

FOR THE STEW
- 1 tbsp rapeseed oil
- 2 medium onions, chopped
- 2 bay leaves
- 4 thyme sprigs, plus extra leaves to serve
- 550g/1lb 4oz chunks of lean braising steak
- 100ml/3½fl oz red wine
- 1½ tbsp plain flour
- 1 tsp English mustard
- 230g can plum tomatoes
- 500ml/18fl oz vegetable stock
- 280g/10oz carrots, halved lengthways and sliced
- 400g/14oz piece butternut squash, deseeded, peeled and cut into chunks
- 140g/5oz chestnut mushrooms, quartered or halved if large

FOR THE DUMPLINGS
- 140g/5oz self-raising flour
- 2 spring onions, ends trimmed, finely chopped
- 3 tbsp chopped parsley
- 2 tbsp rapeseed oil
- ½ tsp English mustard
- 100ml/3½fl oz buttermilk or a mix of yogurt and milk

1 Heat the oil in a large pan, tip in the onions, bay leaves and thyme sprigs and fry for about 8 mins, stirring often, until the onions are turning golden. Raise the heat, add the steak and stir-fry briefly until it starts to brown. Pour in the wine, stir to deglaze the brown sticky bits from the bottom of the pan, and let it bubble briefly. Lower the heat, sprinkle in the flour and mustard and stir for 1 min. The meat should now be coated in a thick, rich sauce.

2 Mix in the tomatoes and stock and bring to the boil. Tip in the carrots, squash and mushrooms, lower the heat, cover and leave to simmer gently for 1 hr 40 mins, stirring occasionally. Uncover and cook for a further 20 mins, still on a gentle simmer, until the meat is very tender. Season with pepper.

3 When the stew is nearly cooked, heat oven to 190C/170C fan/gas 5. Put a 2.25-litre casserole dish in to heat it up. Meanwhile, make the dumplings. Put the flour in a bowl, then stir in the spring onions and parsley. Mix the oil, mustard and buttermilk together and gently stir into the flour. Add a drop or two of cold water, if needed, to pick up any dry bits on the bottom of the bowl, and stir to make a soft and slightly sticky dough. Be as light-handed as you can, otherwise you will toughen the dumplings. Cut the dough into 8 pieces and very lightly shape each into a rough ball.

4 Carefully transfer the stew to the hot casserole dish and remove the bay leaves and thyme sprigs. Sit the dumplings on top and press them down into the gravy to very slightly submerge. Put the dish on a baking sheet and cook in the oven for about 20 mins until the dumplings have risen and are golden on top. Serve with a light scattering of thyme leaves.

PER SERVING 571 kcals, fat 18g, saturates 4g, carbs 54g, sugars 18g, fibre 9g, protein 38g, salt 0.9g

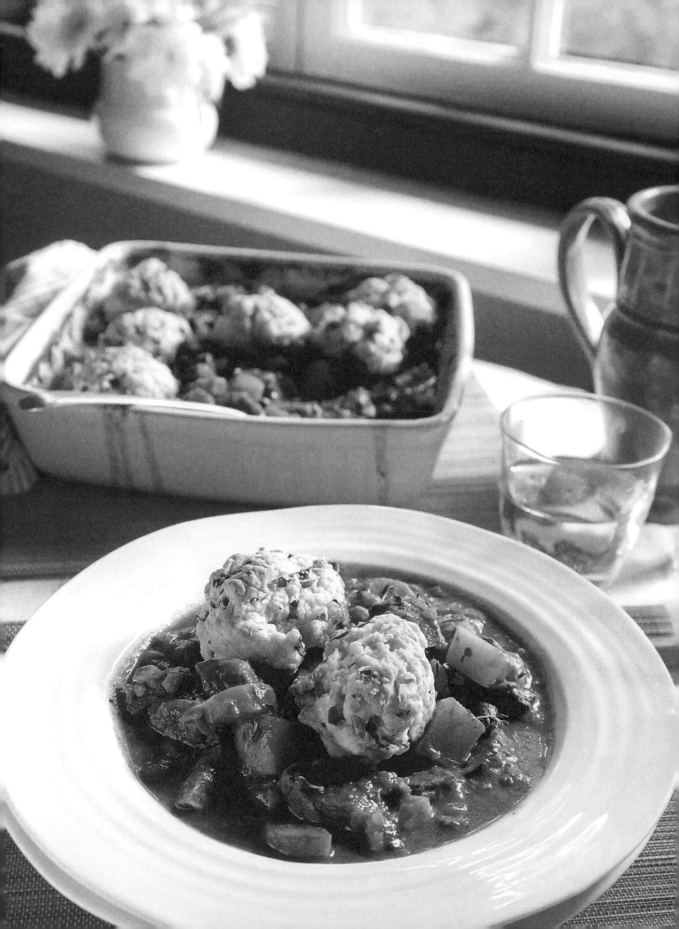

Sloppy Beef Goulash

This low-fat meal in a bowl is like a chunky soup perfect for eating with a spoon. Packed with 3 of your 5 a day it is really satisfying as well as being rich in vitamin C.

🕐 1 hour 5 mins   ◔ 2-3

- 1 tbsp rapeseed oil
- 1 large onion, halved and sliced
- 3 garlic cloves, sliced
- 200g/7oz lean stewing beef, finely diced
- 1 tsp caraway seeds
- 2 tsp smoked paprika
- 400g can chopped tomatoes
- 600ml/1 pint beef stock
- 1 medium sweet potato, peeled and diced
- 1 green pepper, deseeded and diced

FOR TOPPING
- 150g pot natural bio yogurt
- good handful chopped parsley

1 Heat the oil in a large pan, add the onion and garlic and fry for 5 mins until starting to colour. Stir in the beef, increase the heat and fry, stirring, to brown it.

2 Add the caraway and paprika, stir well then tip in the tomatoes and stock. Cover and leave to cook gently for 30 mins.

3 Stir in the sweet potato, and green pepper, cover the pan again and cook for 20 mins more or until tender. Allow to cool a little then serve topped with the yogurt and parsley.

PER SERVING (3) 345 kcals, fat 12g, saturates 4g, carbs 28g, sugars 18g, fibre 7g, protein 25g, salt 1g

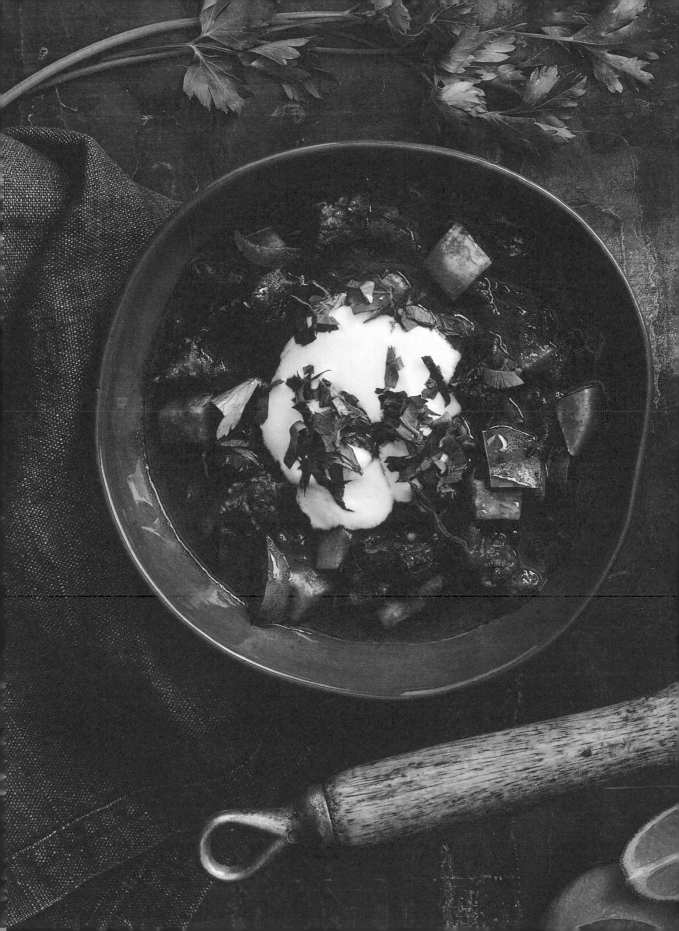

Ginger Beef Lettuce Wraps

These are a bit like healthy spring rolls! Lettuce leaves are used as cups to wrap round the tasty filling. Eat with your fingers for a different supper the family will have fun sharing.

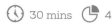 30 mins   4

- 1 tbsp sesame oil
- 200g/7oz lean beef mince
- 8 spring onions, sliced on an angle, green parts reserved
- 1 red pepper, deseeded and chopped
- thumb-sized piece ginger, peeled and finely grated
- 100ml/3½fl oz oyster or hoisin sauce
- 350g/12oz frozen soya beans
- 300g pack cooked rice noodles
- 2 limes, 1 juiced, and 1 cut into wedges
- 2 butter lettuces or 1 iceberg

1 Heat the oil in a non-stick frying pan. Add the beef and fry until browned all over and starting to crisp. Add the spring onions, pepper, ginger, oyster or hoisin sauce and beans. Stir-fry for another 5 mins until the veg has softened, then add the noodles and juice of 1 lime. Season well and toss everything together until well combined and heated through.

2 Separate the lettuces into leaves. Pile the noodles into the leaves, sprinkle over the reserved spring onions to garnish and serve with the lime wedges.

PER SERVING 383 kcals, fat 16g, saturates 4g, carbs 32g, sugars 7g, fibre 8g, protein 23g, salt 2.8g

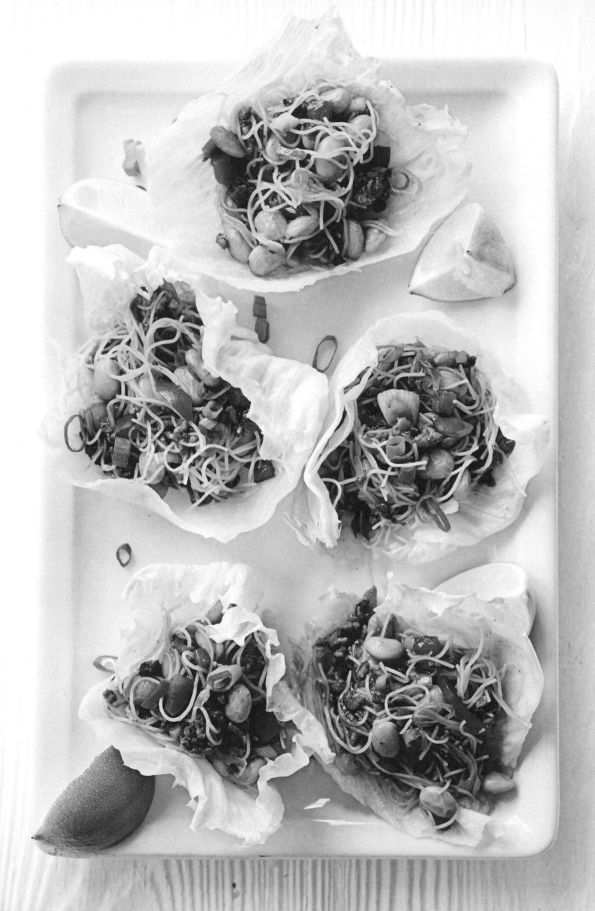

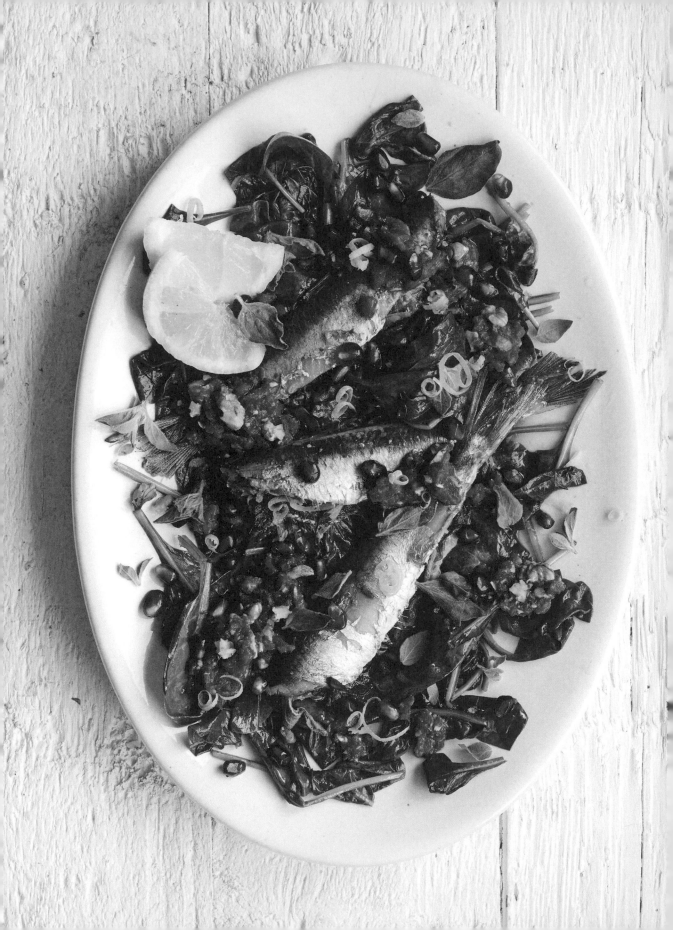

Chapter 4:

FISH & SEAFOOD SUPPERS

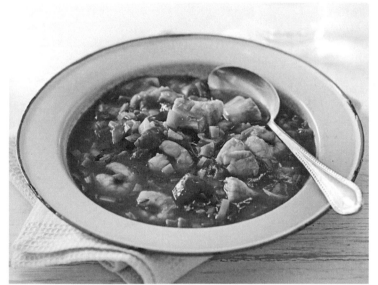

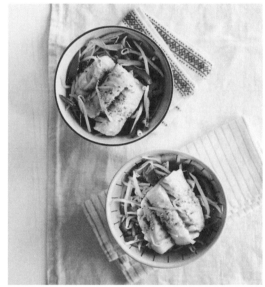

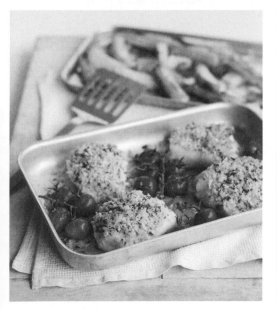

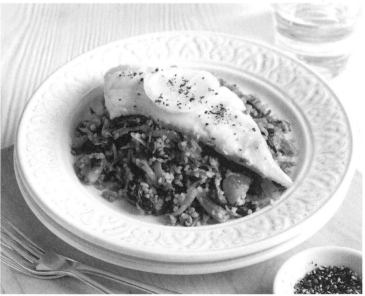

Mackerel with Sizzling Ginger, Garlic & Tomatoes

The omega 3 oils in oily fish are so beneficial for heart health it's recommended that we eat it at least once a week. Mackerel, herrings and sardines are excellent, budget-friendly sources.

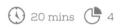 20 mins 4

- 2 large whole mackerel, gutted and cleaned (ask your fishmonger to do this)
- 2 tbsp sunflower or groundnut oil
- thumb-size piece ginger, finely shredded
- 3 garlic cloves, thinly sliced
- 2 fat red chillies, deseeded and shredded
- bunch spring onions, finely shredded
- 250g/9oz cherry tomatoes
- 1 tsp white wine vinegar
- 1 tbsp soy sauce, preferably reduced-salt, plus extra to serve

1 Heat the grill to high or fire up the bbq. Slash the fish a few times on each side, then season with black pepper. Grill or barbecue the fish for 3–5 mins each side until charred and cooked through. The flesh should flake easily when tested with a knife.

2 Heat the oil in a frying pan (you can put it on the barbecue rack) then fry the ginger, garlic and chillies for about 2 mins until the garlic is lightly golden, Take off the heat and toss in the spring onions and tomatoes. Lift the fish on to a plate, splash with the vinegar, then spoon over the contents of the pan and splash with soy sauce. Serve half a fish per person.

PER SERVING 293 kcals, fat 22g, saturates 4g, carbs 3g, sugars 3g, fibre 1g, protein 20g, salt 0.9g

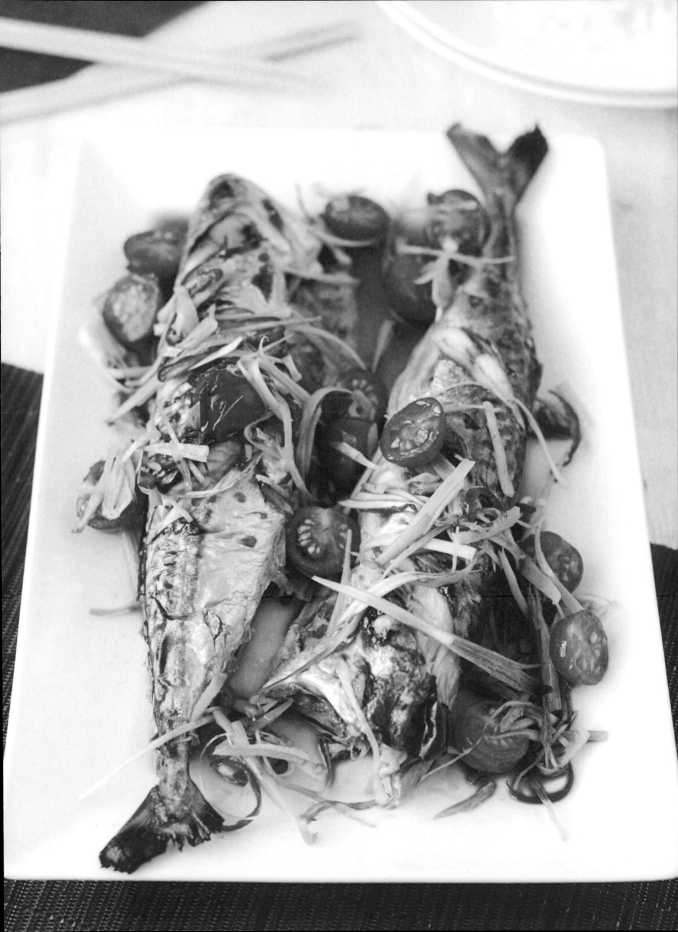

Apple & Beet Salad with Horseradish Mackerel Cream

Smoked mackerel has healthy omega 3 oils, but the smoking process makes it quite salty so eat it in moderation. Here the fish is combined with crisp apples, horseradish and beetroot.

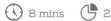 8 mins   2

- 2 red-skinned apples, peel left on, cored and diced
- squeeze lemon (optional)
- good handful mixed salad leaves
- 6 cooked baby beets, plain or spicy, halved or quartered
- 100g/4oz smoked mackerel, flaked
- 150g pot 0%-fat bio yogurt
- 2 tsp hot horseradish sauce
- 2 tbsp sunflower seeds or mixed seeds
- good snipping fresh dill

1 If you are not eating this straight away, toss the apple in a little lemon to stop it going brown. Pile the salad leaves into a container or bowl then top with the apple and beets.

2 Mix the mackerel with the yogurt and horseradish sauce to make an almost mousse-like consistency. Spoon the mackerel onto the salad, and scatter with the seeds and dill.

PER SERVING 418 kcals, fat 24g, saturates 4g, carbs 31g, sugars 26g, fibre 7g, protein 20g, salt 1.5g

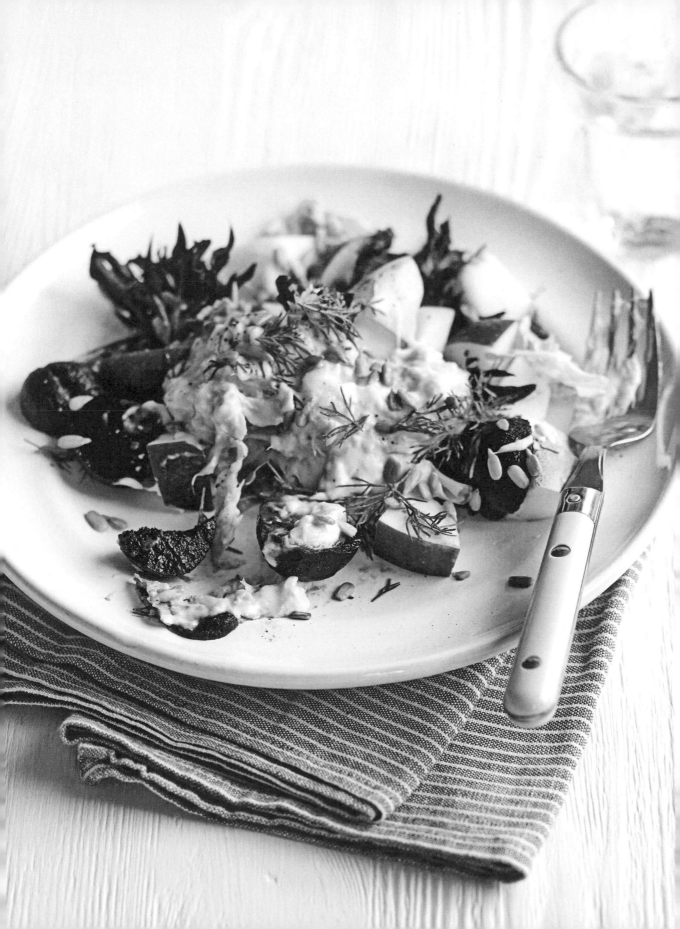

Lemon Sardines with Walnut & Pepper Dressing

The ready boned butterflied fillets from the freezer cabinet couldn't be easier to prepare and eat in this salad, which includes 3 of your 5 a day.

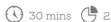 30 mins 2

- 6 butterflied sardines, thawed if frozen
- 2 garlic cloves, finely grated
- juice and zest 1 lemon
- 2 tsp fresh oregano or 1 tsp soft thyme leaves, plus a few extra leaves for sprinkling
- 6 walnut halves
- 100g/4oz roasted red peppers from a jar (not in oil)
- small drizzle of rapeseed oil
- 175g/6oz baby spinach leaves
- the seeds from ½ a pomegranate

1 Open up the sardines and smear the flesh with half the garlic then grate over the lemon zest (reserving a little to serve) and season with black pepper. Scatter over half the herbs then fold the fish in half to reshape them.

2 Put the walnuts, remaining herbs and the peppers in a bowl then blitz to a rough purée with a hand blender. Add the remaining garlic and a generous squeeze of lemon from half of it then blitz again.

3 Rub a large non-stick frying pan with a little oil and heat a drop in a wok, then cook the sardines for 2 mins each side in the frying pan and quickly wilt the spinach in the wok. Arrange the spinach on 2 plates and top with the sardines, scatter over the pomegranate then top with the dressing. Sprinkle over the reserved lemon zest and a few herb leaves, then serve with the remaining half of the lemon, cut into wedges.

PER SERVING 335 kcals, fat 17g, saturates 3g, carbs 14g, sugars 10g, fibre 6g, protein 27g, salt 0.7g

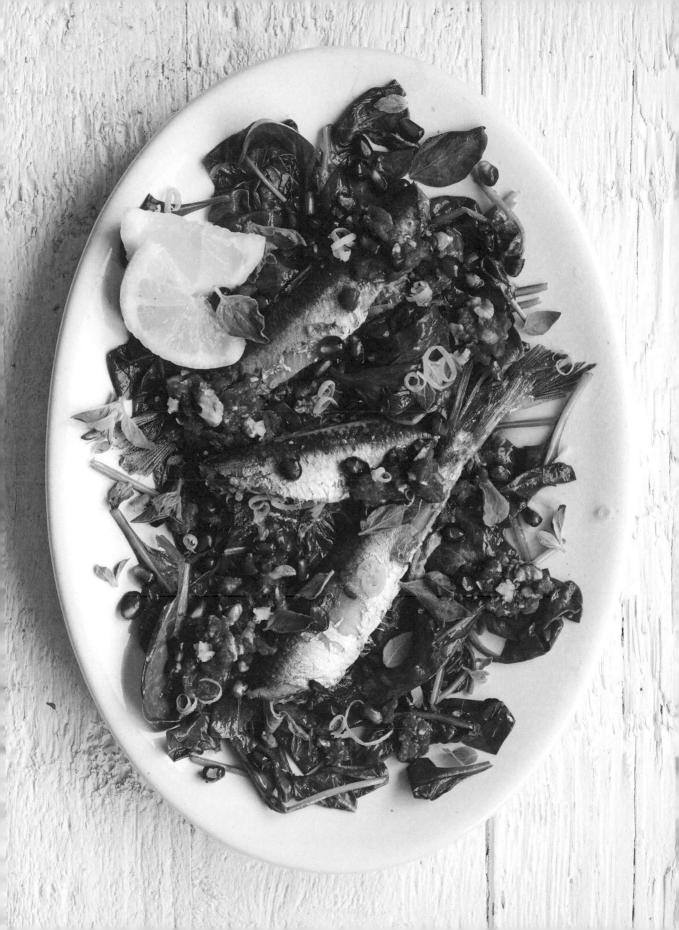

Salsa Spaghetti with Sardines

Canned sardines are a quick, easy way to eat oily fish so we've tossed them through pasta with the robust flavours of olive, lemon and chilli. They are also a delicious snack on toast.

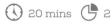 20 mins 2

- 100g/4oz wholewheat spaghetti
- 2 large ripe tomatoes, finely chopped
- 1 red onion, very finely chopped
- 15g/½oz pitted kalamata olives, quartered or 1–2 tbsp capers
- ½ tsp finely chopped red chilli
- ½ lemon, grated zest and juice to taste
- 4 tbsp shredded basil
- 2 x 120g cans sardines in olive oil, drained and oil reserved (optional)

1 Cook the spaghetti according to the pack instructions. Meanwhile, mix the tomatoes with the onion, olives, chilli, lemon zest and basil. Heat the sardines either in the microwave or in a pan.

2 Drain the pasta, return to the pan and toss with the tomato mixture. Add the sardines in chunky pieces. Season with lemon juice, pepper and a little oil from the tin, if you like.

PER SERVING 442 kcals, fat 16g, saturates 3g, carbs 43g, sugars 10g, fibre 7g, protein 31g, salt 1.7g

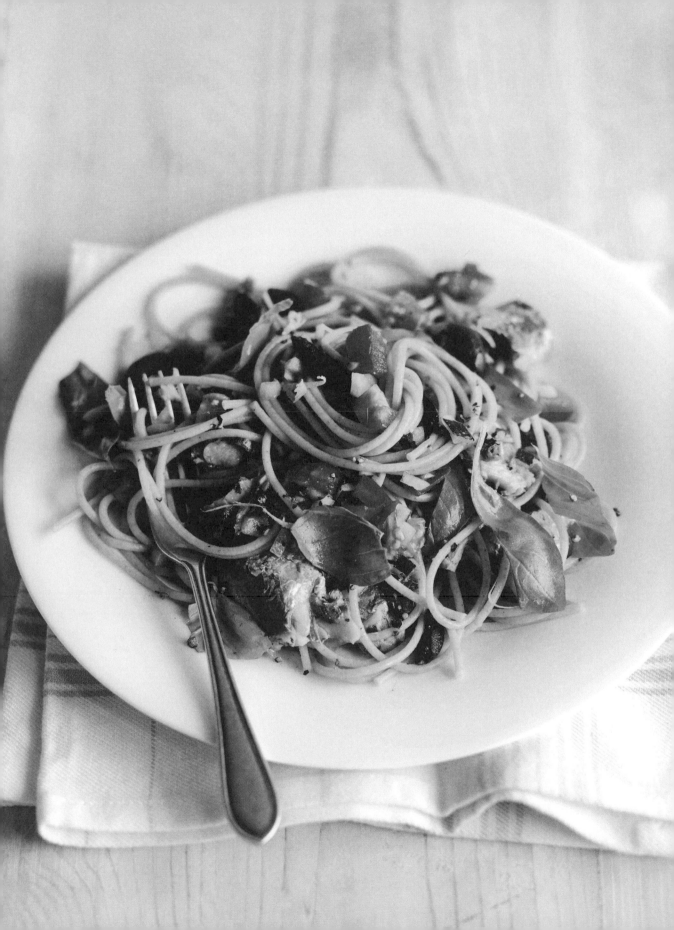

Lemon Pollock with Sweet Potato Chips

Frozen pollock fillets are really good value and are usually just labelled 'white fish fillets' in supermarkets. Served with sweet potato chips and a veg crush this provides 3 of your 5 a day.

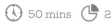 50 mins 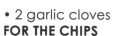 2

- 2 garlic cloves

FOR THE CHIPS
- 2 sweet potatoes, scrubbed and cut into chips
- 2 tsp olive oil
- ½ tsp smoked paprika

FOR THE FISH & DRESSING
- 2 pollock fillets (about 100g/4oz each)
- 2 tbsp olive oil
- zest ½ lemon
- 1½ tsp capers, rinsed and chopped
- 1 tbsp chopped dill

FOR THE BROCCOLI MASH
- 1 leek, chopped
- 4 broccoli spears (about 200g/7oz)
- 85g/3oz frozen peas
- handful mint

1 Heat oven to 200C/180C fan/gas 6. Finely chop the garlic, put half in a bowl for the dressing and set the rest aside for the chips. Toss the sweet potatoes with the oil and spread out on a large baking sheet. Bake for 25 mins, turning halfway through.

2 Put the fish on a sheet of baking parchment on a baking sheet, brush with a little oil, then grate over the lemon zest and season with black pepper. Set aside.

3 Boil the leek for 5 mins, then add the broccoli and cook for 5 mins more. Tip in the peas for a further 2 mins. Drain, return them to the pan and blitz with a hand-held blender to make a thick purée. Add the mint, then blitz again.

4 Meanwhile, toss the reserved garlic and paprika with the chips and return to the oven with the fish for 10 mins. Add the olive oil to the garlic reserved for the dressing, with the capers and dill and 1 tbsp water. Serve everything together with the caper dressing spooned over the fish.

PER SERVING 531 kcals, fat 18g, saturates 3g, carbs 55g, sugars 28g, fibre 16g, protein 30g, salt 0.6g

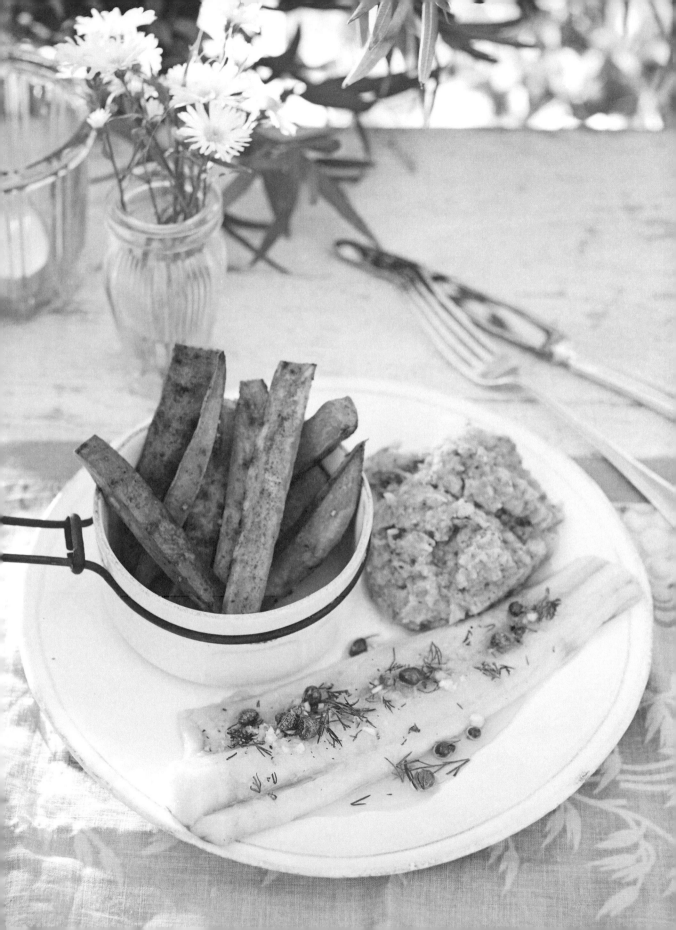

Red Spiced Fish with Green Salad

Spice and herb pastes are amazing for adding lots of flavour with the minimum of effort. For a herby version use pesto with basil leaves instead of coriander.

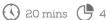 20 mins 4

- 4 fillets white fish, such as pollock or cod
- 4 tsp Thai red curry paste
- 1 avocado, halved, stoned and sliced
- 1 cucumber, sliced into fingers
- 1 romaine or 2 Little Gem lettuces, leaves separated
- small bunch coriander, roughly chopped
- zest and juice 1 lime, plus extra wedges to serve
- 1 tsp clear honey
- 250g/9oz brown rice, cooked, to serve

1 Heat oven to 200C/180C fan/gas 6. Brush each fish fillet with 1 tsp of curry paste, then roast on a baking sheet for 8–10 mins until the fish flakes easily.

2 Meanwhile, mix together the rest of the ingredients, apart from the rice, in a large bowl with some seasoning. Serve with the spiced fish and brown rice, with some extra lime wedges for squeezing over.

PER SERVING 221 kcals, fat 10g, saturates 2g, carbs 4g, sugars 3g, fibre 2g, protein 29g, salt 0.67g

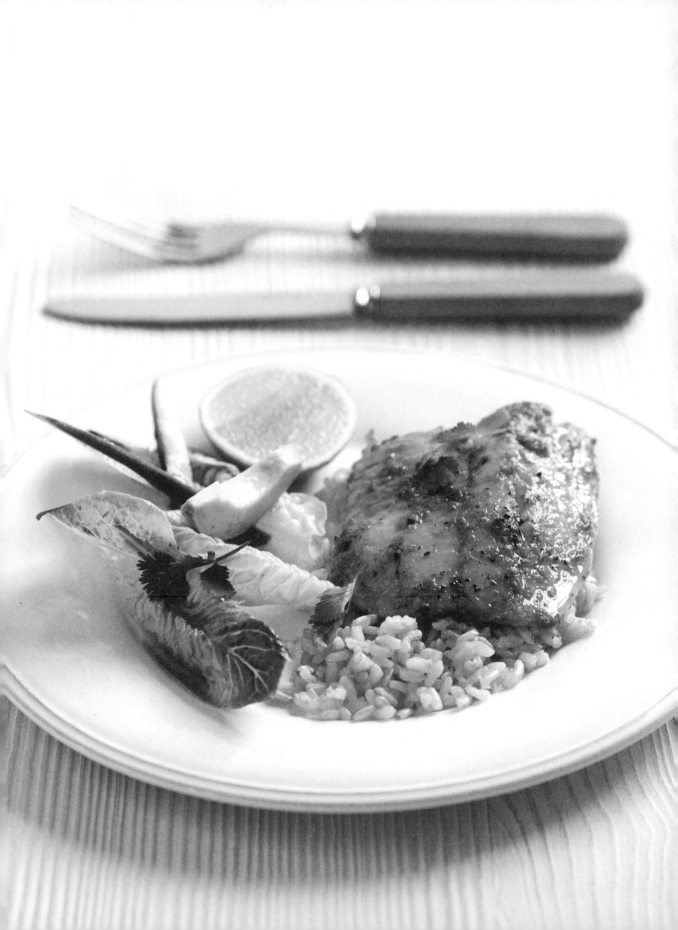

Spiced Bulghar Pilaf with White Fish

Bulghar wheat is a very versatile grain, ideal as an alternative to rice and excellent for absorbing flavours. You can soak it and use it as a base for salads, too.

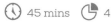 45 mins 4

- 1 tbsp olive oil
- 2 onions, finely sliced
- 3 carrots, grated
- 2 tsp cumin seeds
- 2 tbsp harissa
- 200g/7oz bulghar wheat
- 6 dried apricots, chopped
- 700ml/1¼ pints weak chicken stock (we used 1 stock cube)
- 200g/7oz baby spinach
- 4 firm white fish fillets
- 4 thin lemon slices

1 Heat the oil in a lidded flameproof casserole dish. Tip in the onions and cook for 10 mins until soft and golden. Add the carrots and cumin seeds and cook for 2 mins more. Stir through the harissa, bulghar and apricots, pour over the stock and bring to the boil. Cover and simmer for 7 mins.

2 Add the spinach and stir through until just wilted. Arrange the fish fillets on top, pop a slice of lemon on each and season. Replace the lid and cook for 8 mins, keeping over a low-ish heat.

3 Turn heat to low and cook for 7–8 mins more until the fish is cooked through and the bulghar is tender. Season with pepper and serve.

PER SERVING 416 kcals, fat 6g, saturates 1g, carbs 52g, sugars 15g, fibre 7g, protein 37g, salt 1.0g

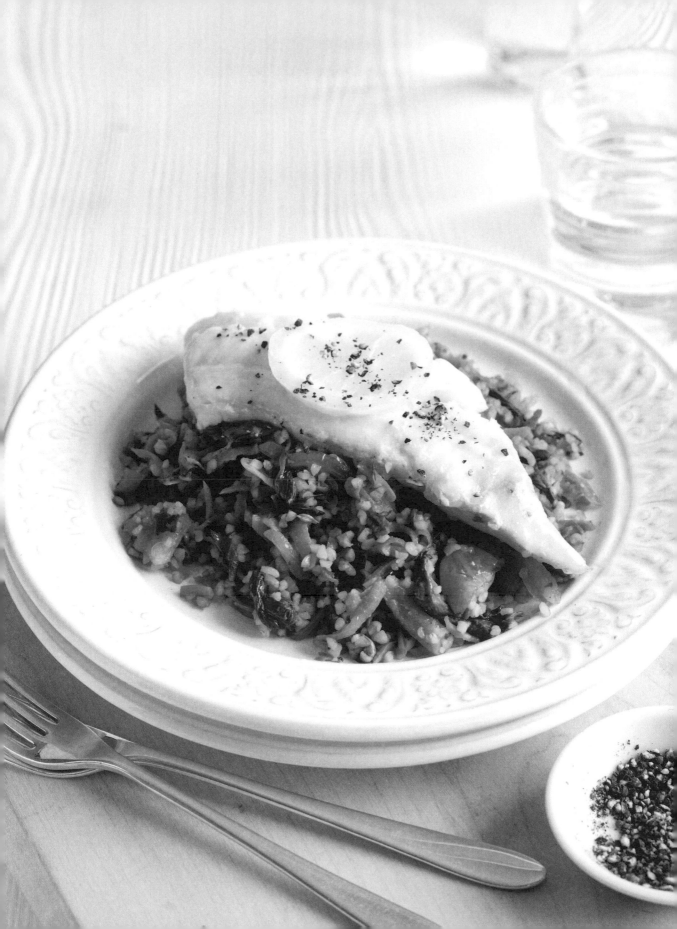

Oven-baked Fish & Chips

This low-fat version of fish and chips couldn't be simpler as they are both baked in the oven. Serve with peas or broccoli.

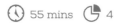 55 mins 4

- 800g/1lb 12oz floury potatoes, scrubbed and cut into chips
- 2 tbsp olive oil
- 50g/2oz fresh breadcrumbs
- zest 1 lemon
- 2 tbsp chopped flat-leaf parsley
- 4 x 140g/5oz thick sustainable white fish fillets
- 200g/7oz cherry tomatoes

1 Heat oven to 220C/200C fan/gas 7. Pat chips dry on kitchen paper, then lay in a single layer on a large baking tray. Drizzle with half the olive oil then cook for 40 mins, turning after 20 mins, so they cook evenly.
2 Mix the breadcrumbs with the lemon zest and parsley, then top the fish evenly with the breadcrumb mixture and drizzle with the remaining oil. Put in a roasting tin with the cherry tomatoes, then bake in the oven for the final 10 mins of the chips' cooking time.

PER SERVING 366 kcals, fat 7g, saturates 1g, carbs 43g, sugars 3g, fibre 4g, protein 32g, salt 0.5g

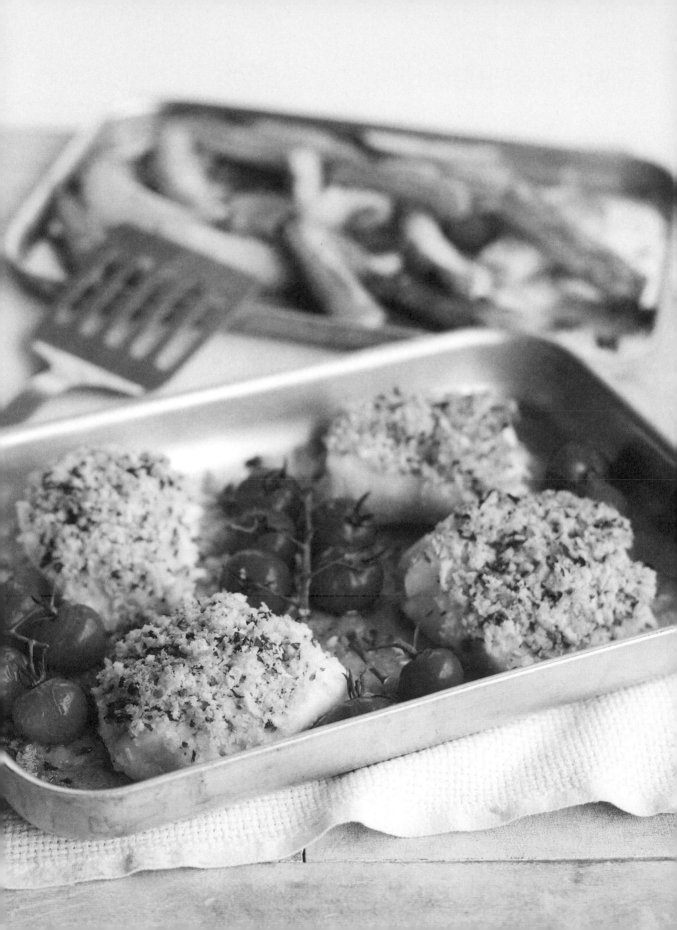

Fish Pie Fillets

Filo adds a crunchy topping to these fish fillets with prawns and soft cheese. Serve with green beans or a salad, with new potatoes in their skins.

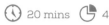 20 mins 4

- 4 x 175g/6oz thick white fish fillets (we used haddock)
- small bunch dill, leaves only, chopped
- 100g/4oz half-fat soft cheese
- 200g/7oz frozen prawns, raw or cooked, defrosted
- 4 sheets filo pastry
- 2 tsp rapeseed oil
- 1 tbsp Parmesan, finely grated

1 Heat oven to 220C/200C fan/gas 7. Put the fish onto a non-stick baking sheet and season all over. Mix the dill and soft cheese in a small bowl, then stir in the prawns, taking care not to break them up. Season with black pepper, then spread evenly over the fish.
2 Brush the filo sheets with the oil, then cut into thick strips. Scrunch the pastry up a little and arrange on top of the fish. Scatter with Parmesan, then bake for 10 mins until the fish is cooked through and the pastry is crisp and golden. (If you've used raw prawns, check they're cooked through.)

PER SERVING 296 kcals, fat 7g, saturates 3g, carbs 13g, sugars 2g, fibre none, protein 46g, salt 1.3g

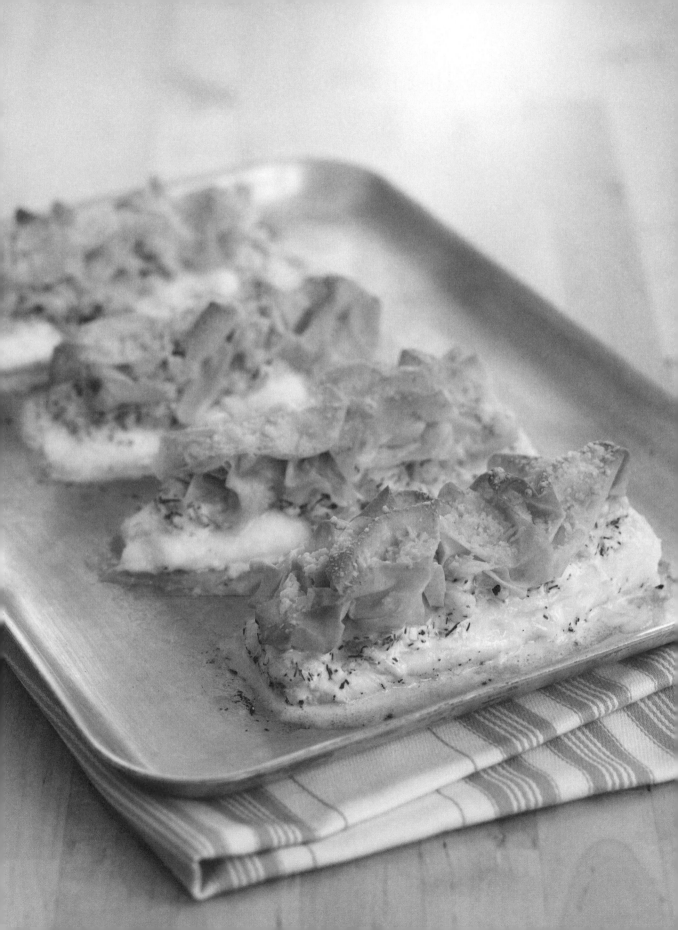

Curry Coconut Fish Parcels

These parcels of sustainable tilapia with curry paste, coconut and lime are steamed in the oven then served with rice and broccoli for a healthy supper.

🕐 20 mins 🥧 2

- 2 large tilapia fillets, about 125g/4½oz each
- 2 tsp red curry paste
- 2 tsp desiccated coconut
- zest and juice 1 lime, plus wedges to serve
- 1 tsp soy sauce, preferably low-salt
- 140g/5oz brown basmati rice
- 2 tbsp sweet chilli sauce
- 1 red chilli, deseeded and sliced
- 200g/7oz cooked thin-stemmed broccoli, to serve

1 Heat oven to 200C/180C fan/gas 6. Tear off 4 large pieces of foil, double them up, then place a fish fillet in the middle of each. Spread over the curry paste. Divide the coconut, lime zest and juice and soy between each fillet. Bring up the sides of the foil, then scrunch the edges and sides together to make 2 sealed parcels.

2 Put the parcels on a baking tray and bake for 10–15 mins. Tip the rice into a pan with plenty of water and boil for 12–15 mins or until cooked. Drain well. Serve the fish on the rice, drizzle over the chilli sauce and scatter with sliced chilli. Serve with broccoli and lime wedges.

PER SERVING 438 kcals, fat 6g, saturates 3g, carbs 63g, sugars 8g, fibre 2g, protein 28g, salt 1.3g

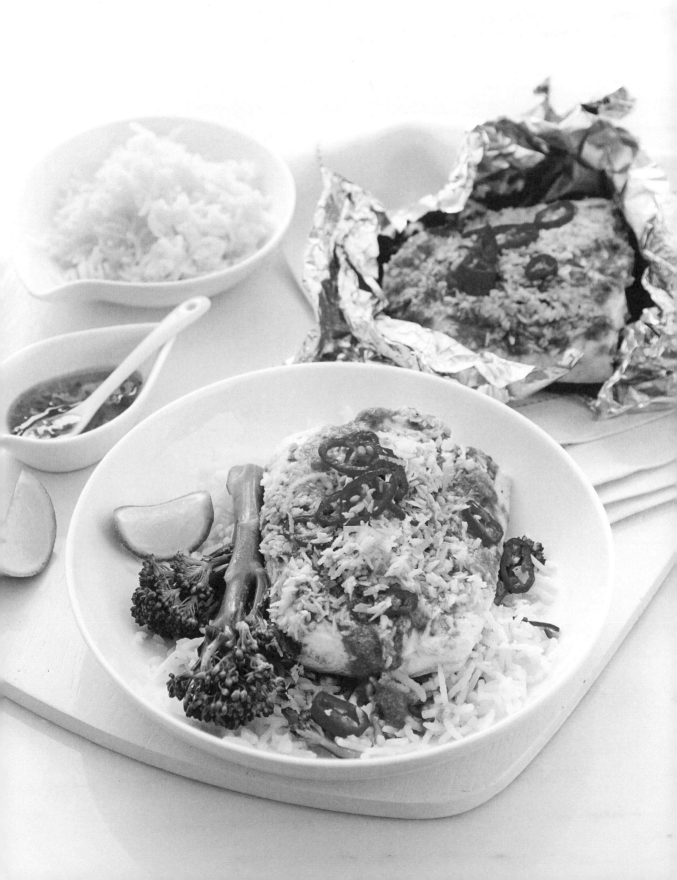

Simple Fish Stew

A quick and healthy low-fat one-pot with white fish and a few prawns and enough veg for 3 of your 5 a day.

🕐 30 mins   🥧 2

- 1 tbsp olive oil
- 1 tsp fennel seeds
- 2 carrots, diced
- 2 celery sticks, diced
- 2 garlic cloves, finely chopped
- 2 leeks, thinly sliced
- 400g can chopped tomatoes
- 500ml/18fl oz hot fish stock
- 2 skinless pollock fillets (about 200g/7oz), thawed if frozen, and cut into chunks
- 85g/3oz raw shelled tiger prawns

1 Heat the oil in a large pan, add the fennel seeds, carrots, celery and garlic and cook for 5 mins until starting to soften. Tip in the leeks, tomatoes and stock, and bring to the boil, then cover and simmer for 15–20 mins until the vegetables are tender and the sauce has thickened and reduced slightly.

2 Add the fish, scatter over the prawns and cook for 2 mins more until lightly cooked. Ladle into bowls and serve.

PER SERVING 346 kcals, fat 8g, saturates 1g, carbs 20g, sugars 17g, fibre 11g, protein 42g, salt 1.7g

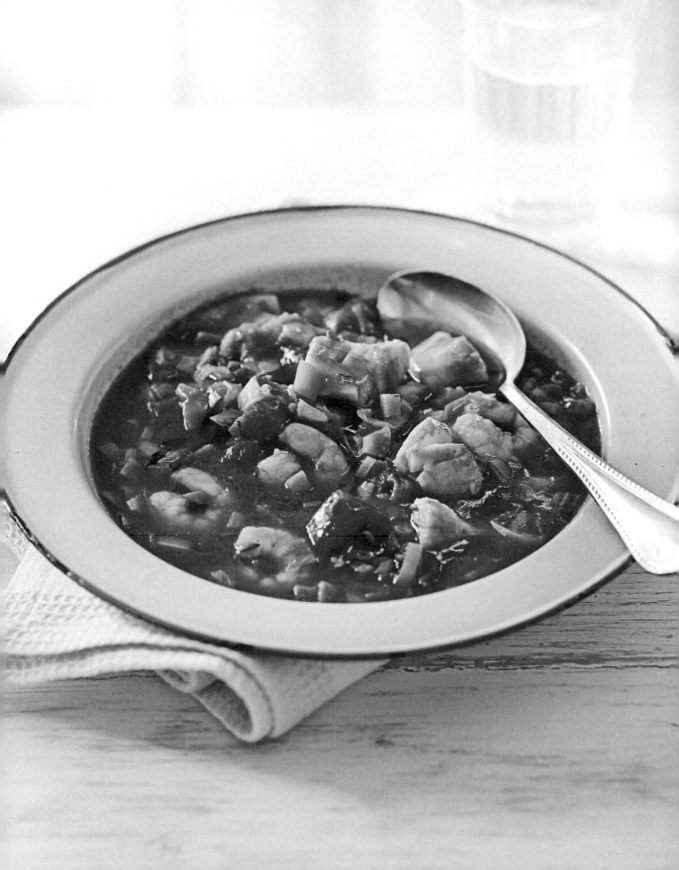

Citrus & Ginger Steamed Fish with Stir-fry Veg

Low-calorie and rich in vitamin C, this speedy supper can be on the table in 20 mins.

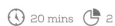 20 mins 2

- 1 orange, grated zest and juice
- 1 tbsp soy sauce, preferably reduced-salt
- 2 tsp white wine vinegar
- 2 skinless white fish fillets
- 1 tbsp very finely shredded ginger
- 2 tsp sesame oil
- 10 spring onions, halved and sliced lengthways
- 2 garlic cloves, thinly sliced
- 1 red pepper, deseeded and thinly sliced
- 150g/5½oz beansprouts
- 1–2 tsp toasted sesame seeds

1 Mix the orange juice and zest with the soy and vinegar. Line the top of a steamer with baking paper and heat the water in the base. Top the fish fillets with a little ginger then arrange them in the steamer, spoon 2 tbsp of the dressing over the fish then cover and steam for 5–6 mins until the fish flakes easily when tested.

2 Meanwhile, heat the sesame oil in a non-stick wok then stir-fry the onions, garlic, pepper and remaining ginger for 2 mins. Add the beansprouts and cook for 2 mins more. Pour any juices from the fish into the vegetables. Stir through the dressing then divide between bowls, top with the fish and scatter with the seeds.

PER SERVING 259 kcals, fat 6g, saturates 1g, carbs 14g, sugars 11g, fibre 5g, protein 33g, salt 1.2g

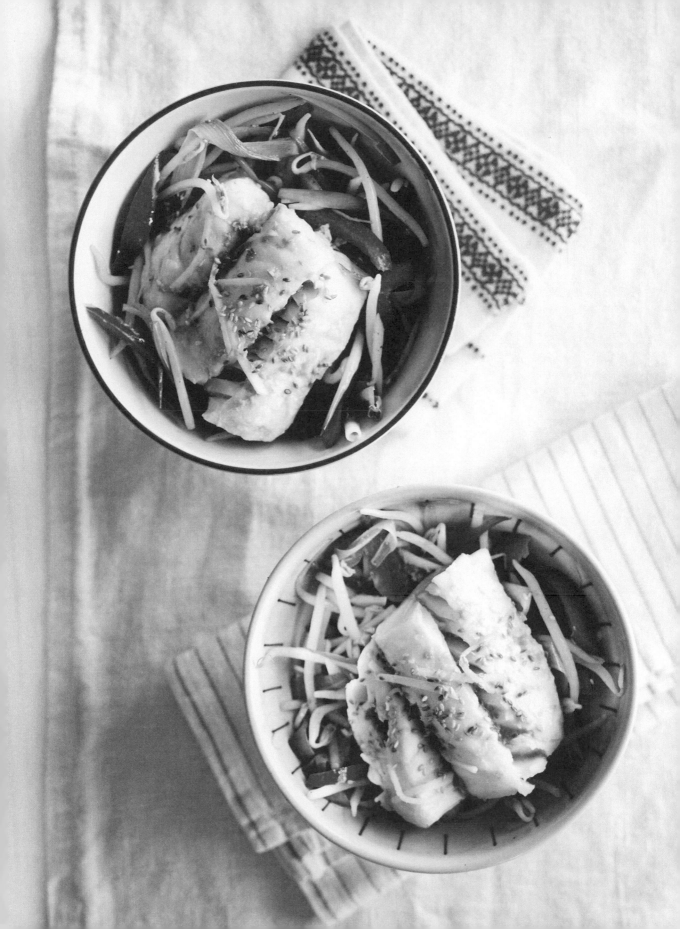

Poached Fish with Ginger & Sesame Broth

Frozen soya beans add to the protein in this subtle-tasting broth that's packed with white fish and vegetables.

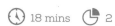 18 mins 2

- 500ml/18fl oz fish stock or weak chicken stock
- 1 tbsp white wine vinegar
- 2–4 slices fresh ginger
- 2 garlic cloves, shredded
- 85g/3oz frozen soya beans or peas
- 100g/4oz Tenderstem broccoli, halved if large
- 4 Chinese leaves, shredded or small pak choi
- 3 spring onions, sliced at an angle
- 2 chunky white fish fillets
- few drops sesame oil
- ½–1 tsp toasted sesame seeds

1 Pour the stock into a deep sauté pan or wok with the vinegar then add the ginger and garlic. Cover and cook for 5 mins to allow the flavours to mingle.
2 Add the soya beans, broccoli and the fleshy part of the Chinese leaves then place the spring onions and fish on top. Cover and cook for 4–5 mins more until it just flakes. Carefully lift the fish off, discard the ginger and stir in the remaining Chinese leaf and the sesame oil. Ladle into bowls, top with the fish and sprinkle with the seeds.

PER SERVING 247 kcals, fat 6g, saturates 1g, carbs 6g, sugars 1g, fibre 5g, protein 40g, salt 0.7g

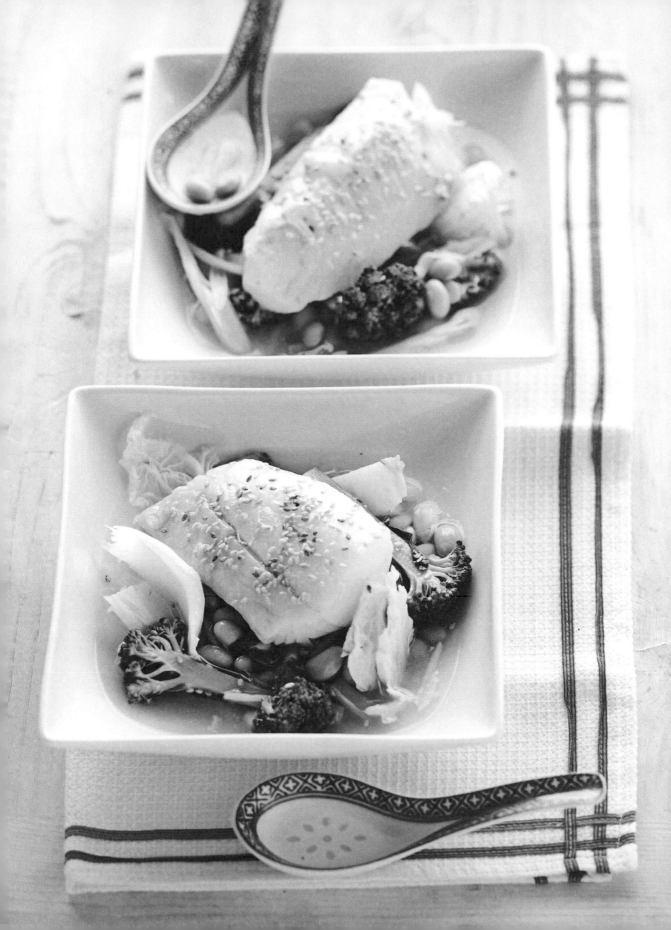

Honey & Lemon Trout with Wilted Spinach

Salmon trout is an oily fish very similar to salmon, which you can use instead, if you prefer.

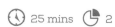 25 mins 2

- small handful thyme sprigs
- 2 salmon trout fillets, skinned
- juice and zest 1 lemon
- 4 tsp rapeseed oil
- 3 garlic cloves, 1 crushed, 2 sliced
- 260g bag baby spinach
- ½ tsp ground nutmeg
- 1–2 tsp clear honey

1 Heat oven to 200C/180C fan/gas 6. Cut 2 large lengths of baking parchment, put thyme in the middle of each one, then top with the trout. Mix the lemon juice with 2 tsp oil and the crushed garlic, pour over the fish and wrap up into 2 parcels, sealing in the juices. Bake for 10 mins on a baking tray.

2 Meanwhile, stir-fry the spinach in 2 tsp oil. When almost wilted, add the garlic and the nutmeg and continue cooking until wilted. Tear the fish parcels open, spoon on the honey and scatter with the lemon zest. Serve still in their parcels, or on top of the spinach.

PER SERVING 333 kcals, fat 17g, saturates 3g, carbs 9g, sugars 8g, fibre 4g, protein 34g, salt 0.5g

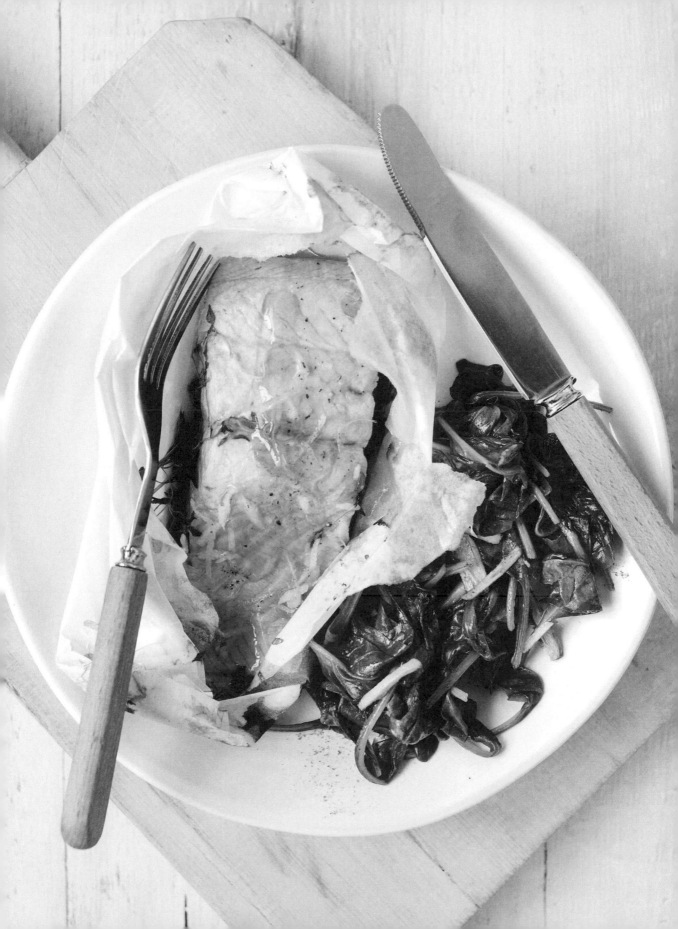

Fish Finger Wraps with Pea Purée

Fish fingers make a quick and easy filling for tortillas – rather than adding tartare sauce, which is high in fat, we have included pea purée.

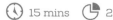 15 mins   2

- 6 fish fingers
- 175g/6oz frozen peas
- ½ tbsp rapeseed oil
- 1 tbsp lemon juice, plus wedges to serve
- 2 wholemeal and seed tortillas
- 2 carrots, coarsely grated
- 1–2 cornichons, sliced
- few rocket leaves (optional)

1. Grill or bake the fish fingers according to the pack instructions. Meanwhile, boil the peas for 3 mins then drain and blitz with the oil and lemon juice with a hand blender (or in a food processor) until smooth. Season, adding a little more lemon, if you like.
2. Warm the tortillas then spread with the pea purée, scatter with the carrot then top with the fish fingers and sliced cornichons. Roll up and eat while still hot and serve with lemon wedges.

PER SERVING 391 kcals, fat 14g, saturates 4g, carbs 43g, sugars 8g, fibre 12g, protein 21g, salt 1.6g

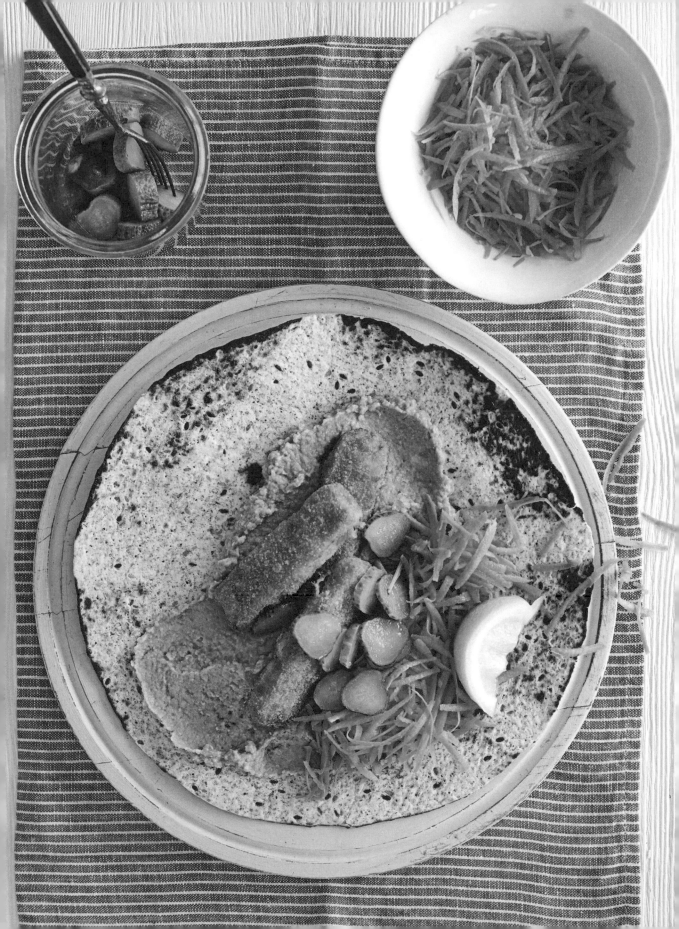

Healthy Salad Niçoise

This French bistro classic makes a filling salad, packed with protein. If you are not a fan of anchovies, swap them for a handful of olives.

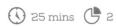 25 mins 2

- 200g/7oz new potatoes, thickly sliced
- 2 medium eggs
- 100g/4oz green beans, trimmed
- 1 romaine lettuce heart, leaves separated and washed
- 8 cherry tomatoes, halved
- 6 anchovies in olive oil, drained well
- 197g can tuna steak in spring water, drained
- 2 tbsp reduced-fat mayonnaise

1 Bring a large pan of water to the boil. Add the potatoes and the eggs and cook for 7 mins. Scoop the eggs out of the pan, tip in the green beans and cook for a further 4 mins. Drain the potatoes, beans and eggs in a colander under cold running water until cool. Leave to dry.

2 Peel the eggs and cut into quarters. Arrange the lettuce leaves in 2 shallow bowls. Scatter over the beans, potatoes, tomatoes and egg quarters. Pat the anchovies with kitchen paper to absorb the excess oil and place on top.

3 Flake the tuna into chunks and scatter over the salad. Mix the mayonnaise and 1 tbsp cold water in a bowl until smooth. Drizzle over the salad and serve.

PER SERVING 351 kcals, fat 17g, saturates 4g, carbs 22g, sugars 6g, fibre 4g, protein 27g, salt 2.1g

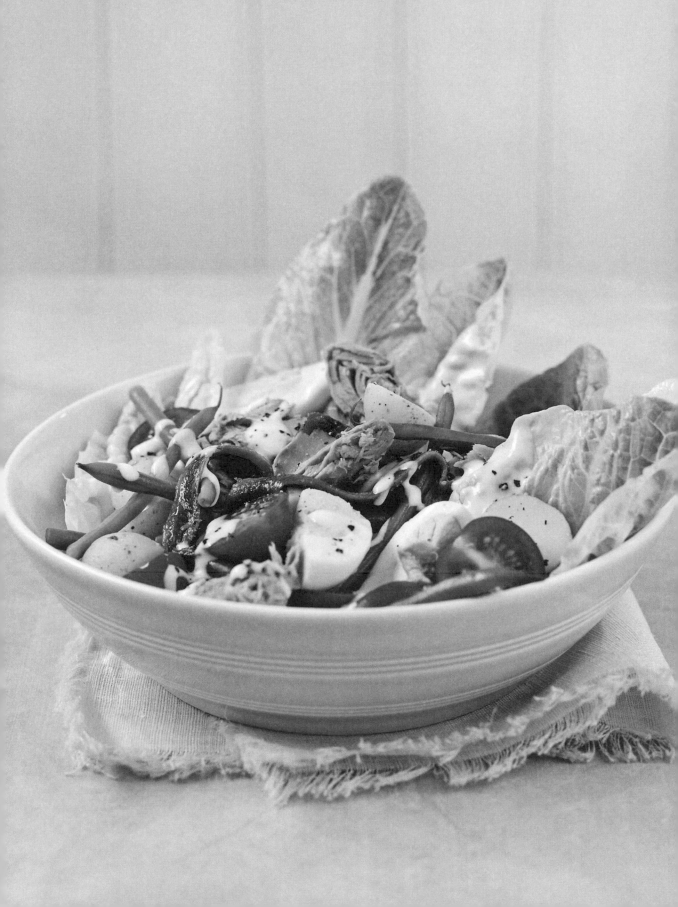

Spaghetti & Tuna Balls

A healthy twist on a family favourite, this recipe uses using tuna to make herby fishballs in a speedy tomato sauce.

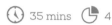 35 mins 4

- 640g can tuna in brine, drained
- 140g/5oz breadcrumbs
- 2 eggs
- 2 tbsp mixed seeds
- ½ small pack tarragon, leaves only, chopped or parsley
- 1 tbsp sunflower oil
- 300g/11oz spaghetti
- 2 x 400g cans cherry tomatoes
- 1 garlic clove, crushed

1 In a large bowl, mix together the tuna, breadcrumbs, eggs, seeds and half of the chopped tarragon. Scrunch the mixture together with your hands and form into golf ball-sized balls.

2 Take a large, deep, non-stick frying pan and add 2 tsp oil. Fry 5–6 balls in the oil over a high heat for 5 mins or until they are a deep golden brown all over, adding more oil if the pan gets dry. Transfer to a plate covered in kitchen paper. Repeat with the rest of the balls.

3 Cook the spaghetti following the pack instructions. Meanwhile, tip the cherry tomatoes into the pan you fried the tuna balls in and add the garlic. Bring to a simmer, then season with black pepper. When the spaghetti has been cooking for a few mins, spoon a ladleful of pasta water into the cherry tomatoes to make a sauce. Just before serving, put the tuna balls back in the pan with the sauce to warm through for 5 mins.

4 Drain the pasta and scatter the remaining tarragon over the tuna balls before serving.

PER SERVING 619 kcals, fat 10g, saturates 2g, carbs 84g, sugars 8g, fibre 5g, protein 45g, salt 1.5g

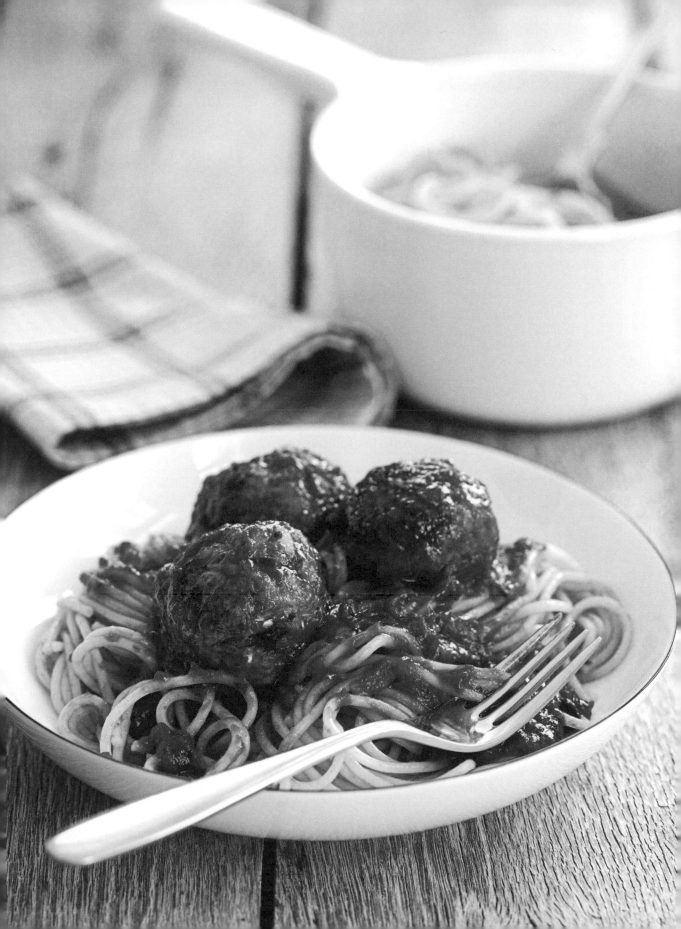

Feelgood Fishcakes with Lemony Mayo

These budget-friendly fishcakes are made with canned sardines – and are perfect for rustling up from just a few ingredients.

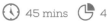 45 mins 4

- 600g/1lb 5oz potatoes, peeled and cut into chunks
- 2 x 120g cans sardines in spring water, drained
- 4 tbsp chopped parsley
- zest and juice 1 small lemon
- 3 tbsp light mayonnaise
- 4 tbsp 0%-fat Greek yogurt
- 1 tbsp plain flour
- 4 tsp rapeseed oil
- green salad and lemon wedges, to serve

1 Boil the potatoes for 15–20 mins until tender. Meanwhile, coarsely mash the sardines in a bowl (there's no need to remove the calcium-rich bones as they are soft enough to eat). Mix in 3 tbsp chopped parsley and half the lemon zest and juice.

2 Stir the mayonnaise and yogurt with the remaining parsley, lemon zest and juice to make the lemony mayo.

3 Drain the potatoes, then mash until smooth. Gently mix into the sardine mixture. Shape into 8 fat fishcakes, then dust lightly with the flour. Chill until ready to cook.

4 Heat half the oil in a non-stick frying pan and fry half the fish cakes for 3–4 mins on each side until golden and crisp. Keep warm while you cook the remaining fishcakes. Serve with the lemony mayonnaise, salad and lemon wedges.

PER SERVING 287 kcals, fat 13g, saturates 2g, carbs 29g, sugars 2g, fibre 2g, protein 16g, salt 0.6g

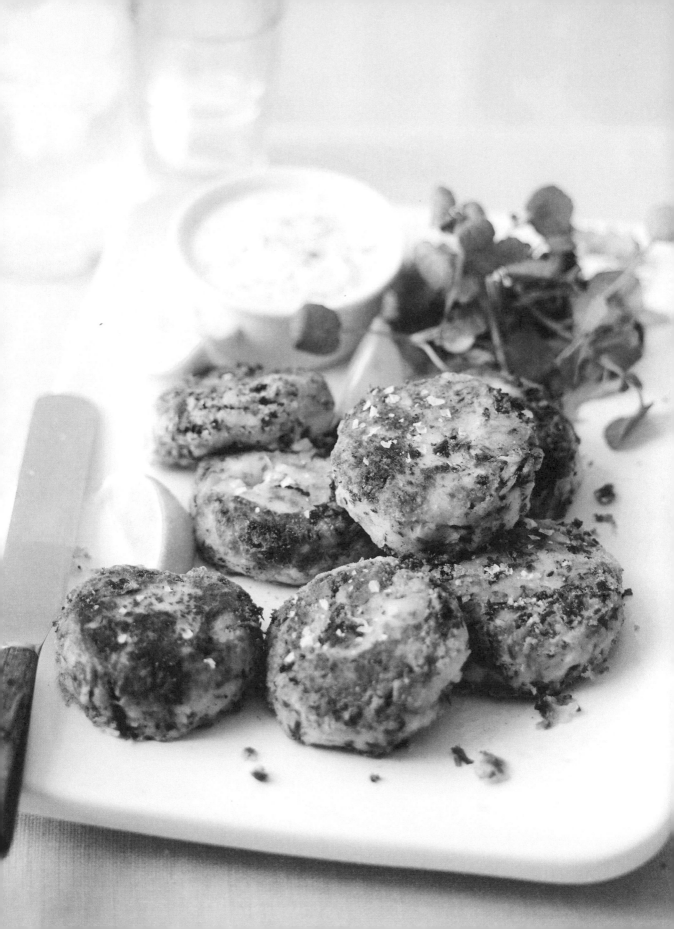

Moroccan Fishcakes

These spicy white-fish-cakes make a lovely supper to eat with a leafy salad. If you like to plan ahead, make up to the end of step 3 then chill, ready to cook and serve.

🕐 1 hour 10 mins   🍴 4

- 600g/1lb 5oz floury potatoes, such as Maris Piper, cut into even chunks
- 300g/11oz skinless and boneless pollock, or other sustainable white fish
- 300ml/½ pint semi-skimmed milk
- 1¼ tsp each paprika and ground cumin
- zest 2 lemons, plus 2 tbsp juice, then cut into wedges to serve
- small pack dill or parsley, leaves finely chopped
- 1 large egg, beaten
- 85g/3oz dried breadcrumbs
- 4 tbsp rapeseed oil, for frying
- 300g/11oz natural yogurt
- 100g bag of salad leaves, to serve

1 Put the potatoes in a saucepan and cover with cold salted water. Bring to the boil and cook for 18–20 mins until cooked but still holding their shape. Drain and leave to steam-dry, then mash.

2 Meanwhile, put the fish in a saucepan and pour over the milk and 100ml water to just cover. Cover with a lid, bring to a simmer, then turn off the heat and leave to finish cooking for 10 mins. Remove the fish with a slotted spoon.

3 Mix 2 tbsp of the poaching milk into the potatoes with 1 tsp each of the spices, the zest of 1 lemon and the dill. Carefully mix the poached fish into the potato, keeping the flakes quite large. Shape into 8 flat fishcakes, then dip each into the beaten egg, then the breadcrumbs.

4 Heat oven to 200C/180C fan/gas 6. Heat the oil in a large non-stick ovenproof frying pan over a medium heat. Add the fishcakes and fry for 5 mins each side until golden and hot through. Transfer to the oven and cook for a further 8–10 mins until piping hot.

5 Meanwhile, mix the yogurt with the remaining lemon zest, 2 tbsp lemon juice and spices. Serve the fishcakes with salad and the sauce.

PER SERVING 477 kcals, fat 18g, saturates 4g, carbs 50g, sugars 11g, fibre 3g, protein 28g, salt 0.9g

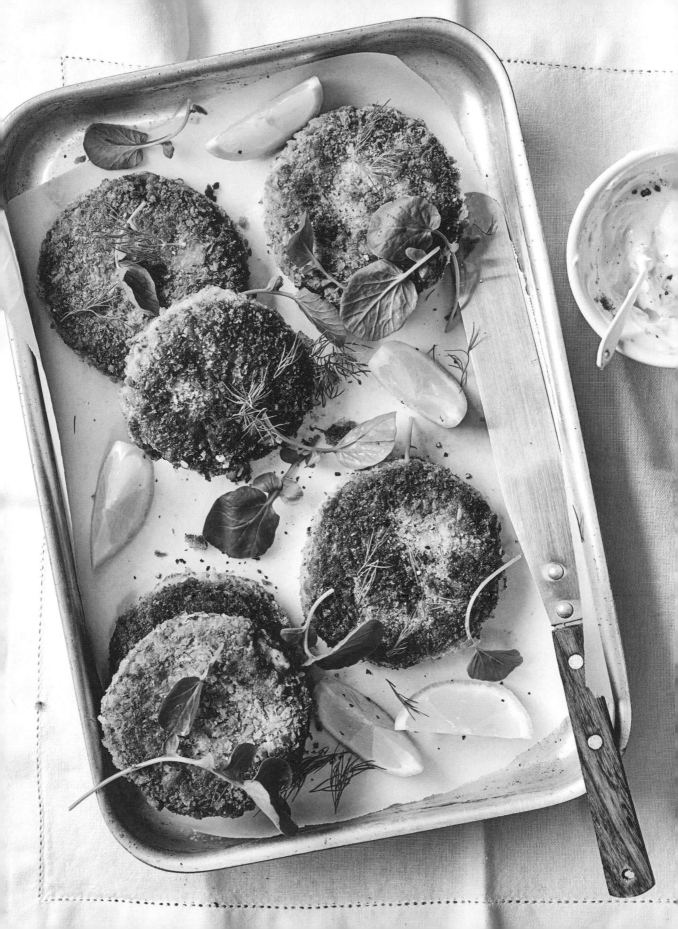

Salmon with Corn & Pepper Salsa Salad

Salmon coated in a spicy Mexican-style rub and served with a chunky salsa for a heart-healthy supper with 3 of your 5 a day.

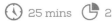 25 mins 2

FOR THE SPICY SALMON
- 1 garlic clove
- ½ tsp mild chilli powder
- ½ tsp ground coriander
- ¼ tsp ground cumin
- 1 lime, grated zest and juice, plus wedges to serve (optional)
- 2 tsp rapeseed oil
- 2 skinless salmon fillets

FOR THE SALSA SALAD
- 1 corn on the cob
- 1 red onion, finely chopped
- 1 avocado, halved, stoned, peeled and finely chopped
- 1 red pepper, deseeded and finely chopped
- 1 red chilli, halved, deseeded and chopped
- ½ pack coriander, finely chopped

1 Finely grate the garlic into a bowl for the spice rub. Boil the corn for the salsa salad for 6–8 mins until tender, then drain and cut off the kernels with a sharp knife.
2 Stir the spices, 1 tablespoon lime juice and the oil into the garlic to make a spice rub, then use to coat the salmon.
3 Mix the remaining lime zest and juice into the corn and stir in all the remaining ingredients. Heat a frying pan and cook the salmon for 2 mins each side so that it is still a little pink in the centre. Serve with the salsa salad with extra lime wedges, if you like, for squeezing over.

PER SERVING 530 kcals, fat 32g, saturates 5g, carbs 27g, sugars 12g, fibre 9g, protein 29g, salt 0.2g

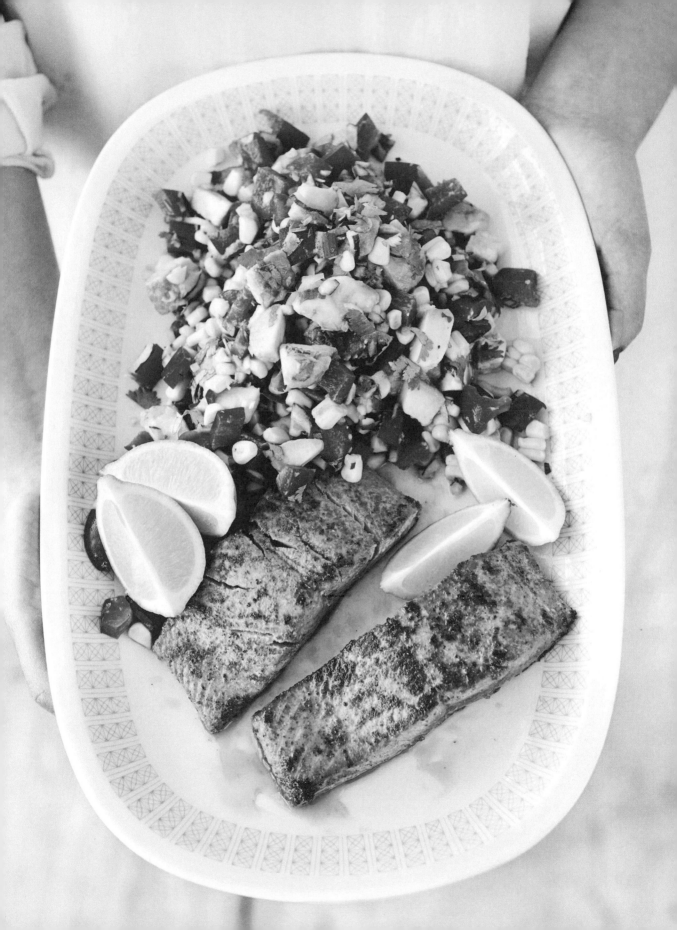

Salmon with Tahini Sauce

Ready in less than 30 mins this healthy supper combines wholewheat couscous with crunchy cucumber and pomegranate.

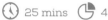 25 mins 4

- 140g/5oz wholewheat couscous
- 4 skinless salmon fillets
- 1 tbsp olive oil
- 4 tbsp tahini
- 2 lemons, 1 juiced, and 1 cut into wedges
- ½ cucumber, chopped into small pieces
- 1 pomegranate, seeds only
- small pack flat-leaf parsley, chopped

1 Tip the couscous into a large heatproof bowl and pour over 400ml boiling water. Cover with cling film and leave to stand for 8–10 mins while you cook the fish.
2 Heat a large, non-stick frying pan over a medium heat. Brush the salmon fillets with olive oil and fry for 5 mins on one side or until opaque halfway up the side of the fillet. Flip the fillets over carefully and cook for another 1–2 mins or until cooked through, then remove from the heat.
3 Mix the tahini with the lemon juice and a splash of water to make a sauce.
4 Drain any excess water from the couscous and tip into a bowl, adding the cucumber, pomegranate seeds and parsley. Serve the salmon on top of the couscous, with lemon wedges on the side and the tahini sauce poured over or served alongside.

PER SERVING 506 kcals, fat 26g, saturates 4g, carbs 31g, sugars 7g, fibre 6g, protein 34g, salt 0.2g

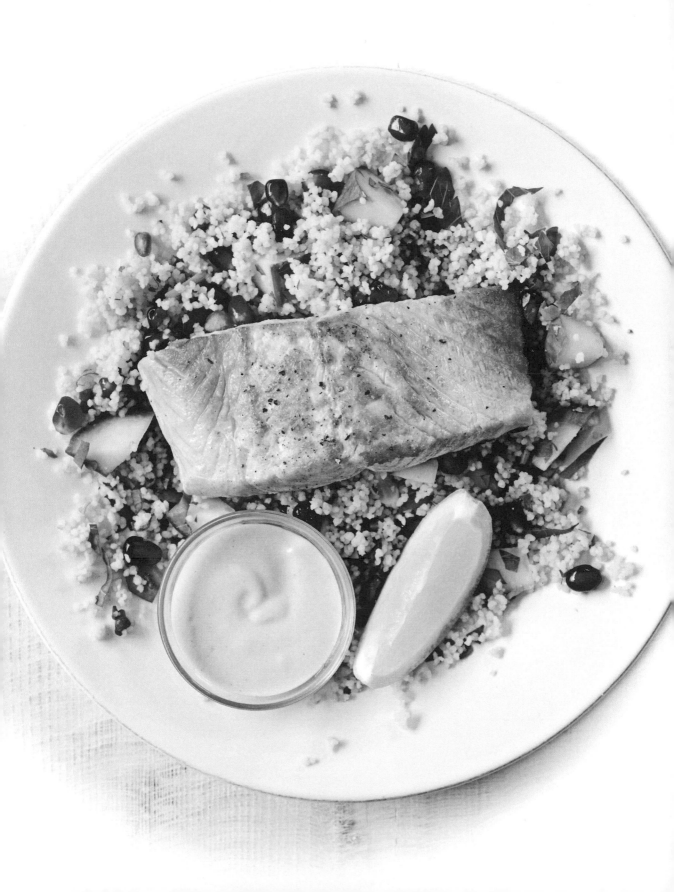

Prawn, Fennel & Rocket Risotto

You can make a small number of prawns go a long way in a dish like this. This is low-fat and low-calorie but has only 1 of your 5 a day, so serve with a generous side salad.

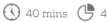 40 mins 4

- 1.2 litres/2 pints vegetable stock
- 1 tbsp olive oil
- 1 onion, finely chopped
- 1 large garlic clove, finely chopped
- 1 small fennel bulb, cored and finely chopped
- 300g/11oz risotto rice
- 300g/11oz raw shelled prawns
- 1 lemon, ½ zested and 1 tbsp juice
- 70g bag rocket

1 Put the stock in a large saucepan, bring to the boil, then lower to a simmer. Meanwhile, heat the oil in a large saucepan. Add the onion, garlic and fennel, and cook on a low heat for 10 mins until the vegetables have softened but not coloured. Add the rice and stir for 2 mins until the grains are hot and making crackling sounds. Increase the heat to medium and start adding the stock, a ladleful at a time, stirring constantly and making sure the stock has been absorbed into the rice before adding the next ladleful.

2 When the rice is almost cooked, add the prawns, lemon zest and some seasoning. Continue adding stock and cooking for another 3–4 mins until the prawns are pink and the rice is cooked. Remove from the heat and stir through the rocket and lemon juice. Check the seasoning, leave the risotto to sit in the pan for 2 mins, then serve.

PER SERVING 391 kcals, fat 5g, saturates 1g, carbs 64g, sugars 5g, fibre 5g, protein 21g, salt 1.2g

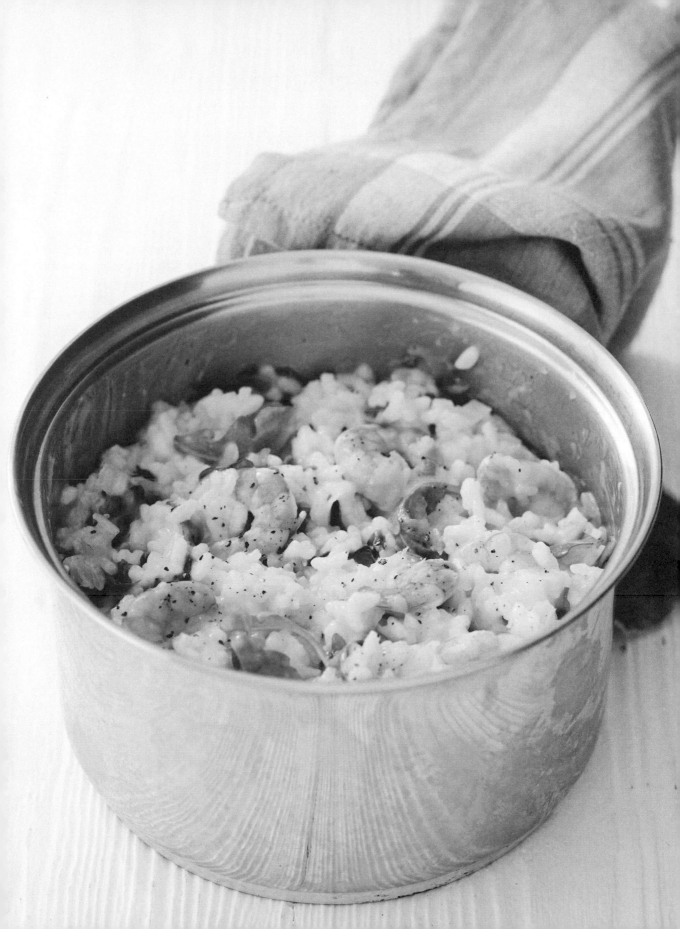

Thai Prawn & Ginger Noodles

If you can't find dried rice noodles, use a pack of the straight-to-wok ones – just skip the soaking stage in the recipe.

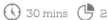 30 mins 2

- 100g/4oz folded rice noodles
- zest and juice 1 small orange
- 1½–2 tbsp red curry paste
- 1–2 tsp fish sauce or soy sauce
- 2 tsp light brown soft sugar
- 1 tbsp rapeseed oil
- 25g/1oz ginger, shredded
- 2 large garlic cloves, sliced
- 1 red pepper, deseeded and sliced
- 85g/3oz sugar snap peas, halved lengthways
- 140g/5oz beansprouts
- 175g pack raw shelled prawns
- handful each chopped basil and coriander

1 Put the noodles in a bowl and pour over boiling water to cover them. Set aside to soak for 10 mins. Stir together the orange juice and zest, curry paste, fish sauce, sugar and 3 tbsp water to make a sauce.

2 Heat the oil in a large wok and add half the ginger and the garlic. Cook, stirring, for 1 min. Add the pepper and stir-fry for 3 mins more. Toss in the sugar snaps, cook briefly, then pour in the curry sauce. Add the beansprouts and prawns and continue cooking until the prawns just turn pink. Drain the noodles, then toss these into the pan with the herbs and remaining ginger. Mix until the noodles are well coated in the sauce, then serve.

PER SERVING 426 kcals, fat 9g, saturates 1g, carbs 59g, sugars 16g, fibre 4g, protein 24g, salt 1.4g

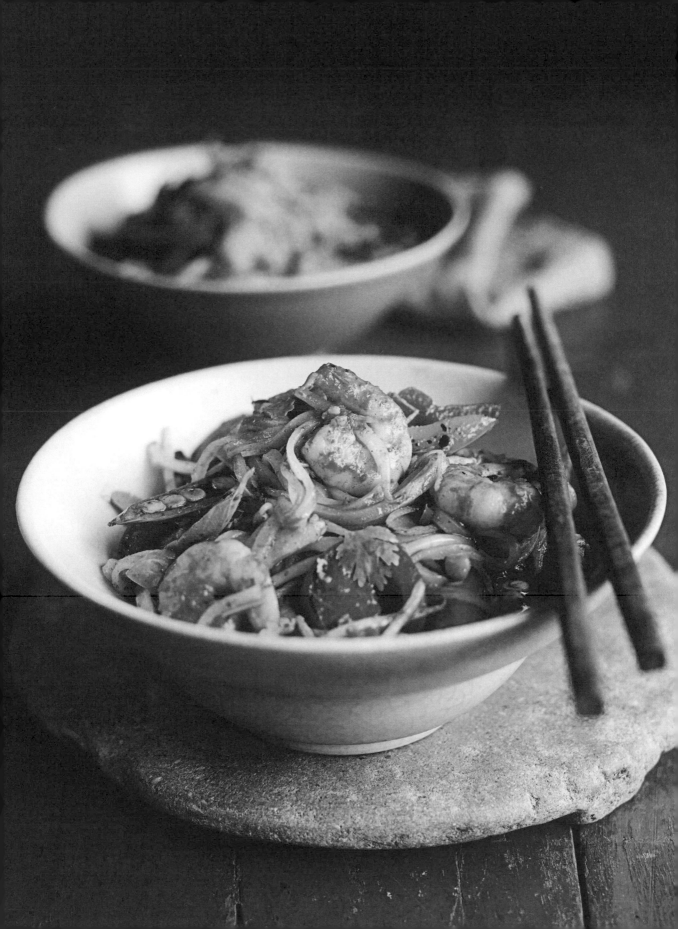

Harissa Prawns with Warm Chickpea Salad

This makes a very speedy supper, packed with good things. You could add some halved cherry tomatoes to the salad, too.

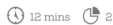 12 mins 2

- 1 tbsp olive oil
- 1 red onion, finely sliced
- 400g can chickpeas, drained
- 50g/2oz shredded curly kale
- 1 tbsp tahini
- juice 1 lemon
- 2 tbsp chopped flat-leaf parsley
- 150g pack raw shelled prawns
- 2 tsp harissa

1 Heat a large non-stick frying pan and add the oil. Tip in the onion and fry over a high heat for 1–2 mins. Add the chickpeas and kale and warm through. Mix the tahini with the lemon juice and parsley, then stir into the pan. Tip onto a serving platter.

2 Return the pan to the heat. Mix the prawns with the harissa and fry for 1–2 mins until the prawns are cooked through. Tip the prawns over the salad and serve.

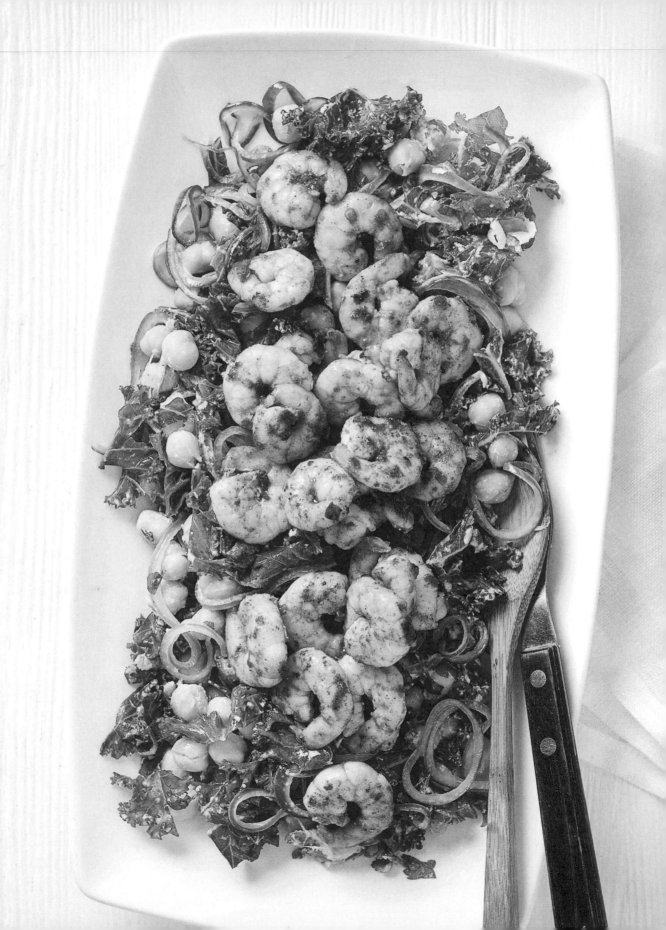

Spaghetti with Smoky Tomato & Seafood Sauce

Seafood may sound luxurious, but the frozen packs are excellent value, and better still they come prepared and ready to use.

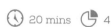 20 mins 4

- 4 tbsp olive oil
- 4 garlic cloves, crushed
- 1 red chilli, deseeded and finely sliced
- 1½ tsp fennel seeds
- 400g/14oz spaghetti
- 2 tsp smoked paprika
- 2 x 400g cans chopped tomatoes
- 400g pack frozen mixed cooked seafood, defrosted
- small bunch parsley or basil, chopped

1 Boil the kettle and heat the oil in a large, deep frying pan. Add the garlic, chilli and fennel seeds, and sizzle for a few mins. Pour the boiling water into a large pan and cook the pasta following the pack instructions.

2 Add the paprika and tomatoes to the pan and simmer for 8-10 mins while the pasta cooks.

3 Drain the pasta 1 min before the end of the cooking time, reserving a cup of the water. Add the pasta to the sauce with the seafood. Simmer for 1–2 mins, adding a splash of the reserved pasta water if it looks too thick. Toss the pasta through the sauce as it cooks. Add the herbs and black pepper, then serve.

PER SERVING 618 kcals, fat 19g, saturates 3g, carbs 80g, sugars 8g, fibre 7g, protein 35g, salt 0.7g

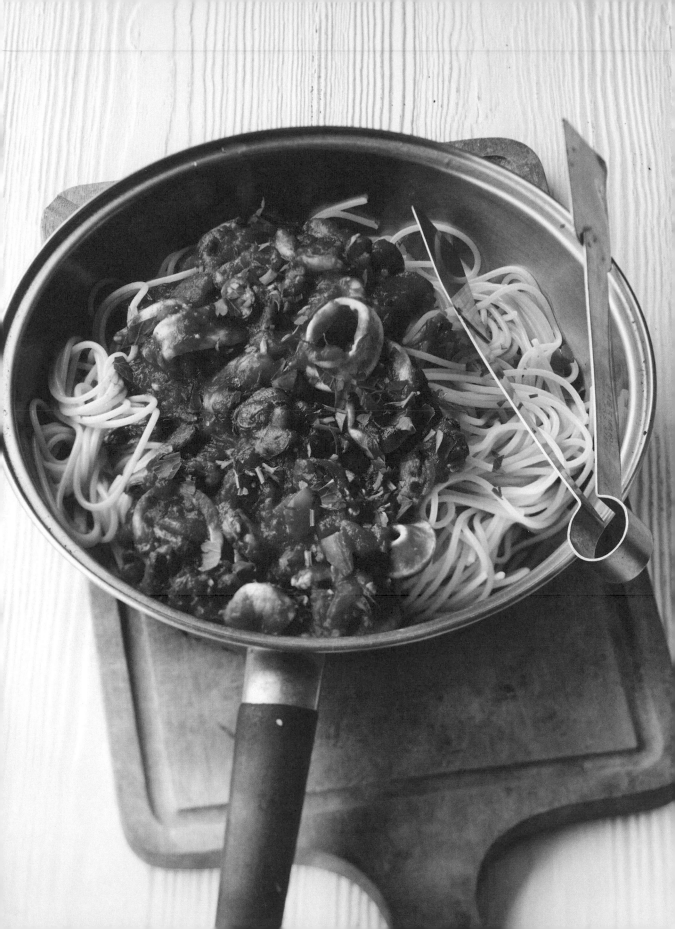

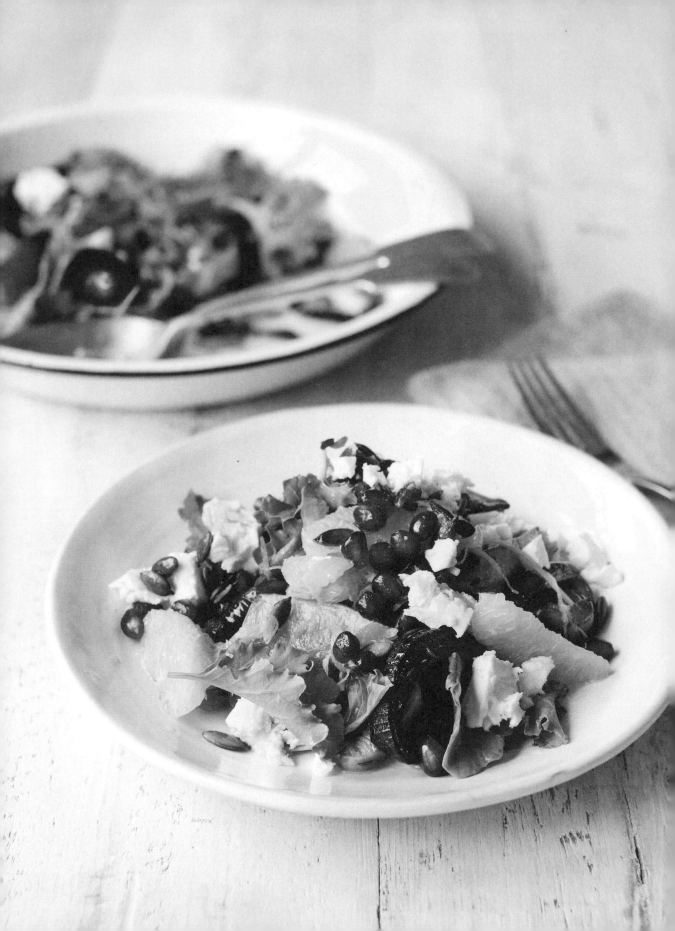

Chapter 5:

MAKE IT VEGETARIAN

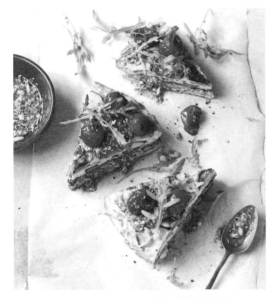

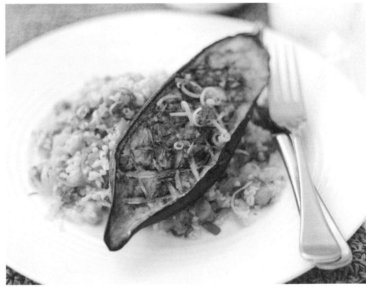

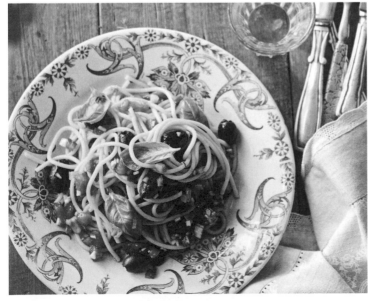

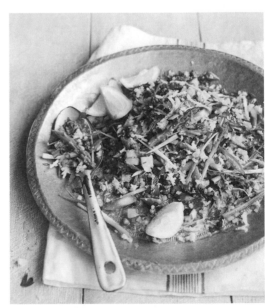

Cauliflower, Paneer & Pea Tikka

Paneer is the cheese used in Indian cuisine. It is firm, mild and doesn't really melt, a bit like halloumi – which you can use instead. This low-fat curry provides 3 of your 5 a day.

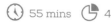 55 mins 4

- 2 tbsp rapeseed oil
- 225g pack paneer, cut into cubes
- 1 cauliflower, broken into small florets
- 2 onions, thickly sliced
- 2 garlic cloves, crushed
- 2 heaped tbsp tikka masala curry paste
- 500g carton passata
- 200g/7oz frozen peas
- small pack coriander, roughly chopped
- rice (preferably brown) or naan, to serve

1 Heat 1 tbsp oil in a large non-stick frying pan, add the paneer and fry gently until crisp. Remove with a slotted spoon and set aside. Add the remaining oil and the cauliflower to the pan and cook for 10 mins until browned. Add the onions and a little more oil, only if needed, and cook for a further 5 mins until softened. Stir in the garlic and curry paste, then pour in the passata and 250ml water. Bring to a simmer, then cover and cook for 18–20 mins or until the cauliflower is just tender.

2 Add the frozen peas and paneer to the pan and cook for a further 5 mins. Stir through most of the coriander and garnish with the rest. Serve with rice or naan.

PER SERVING 321 kcals, fat 14g, saturates 4g, carbs 21g, sugars 15g, fibre 9g, protein 23g, salt 0.4g

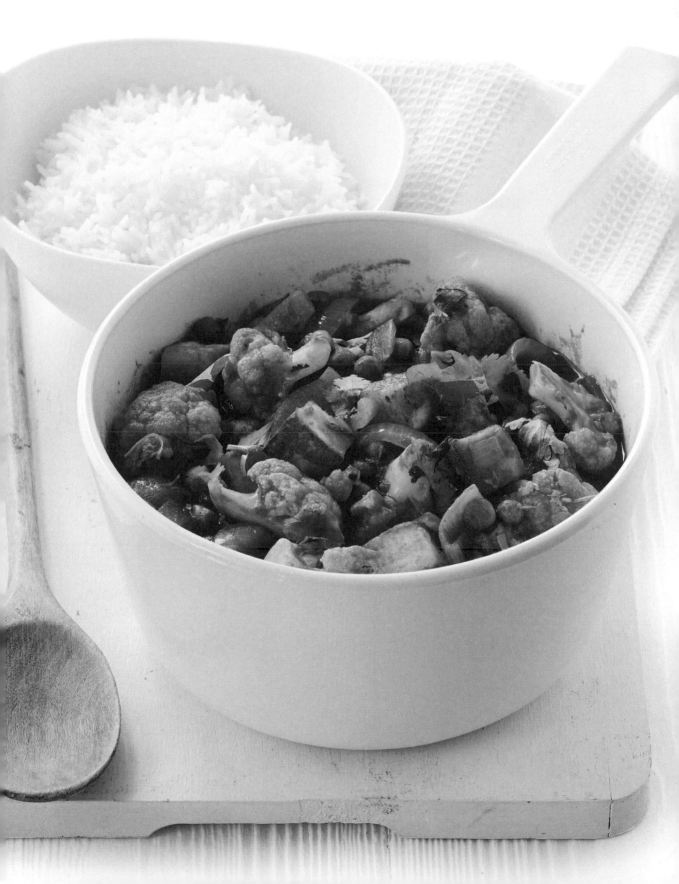

Red Lentil & Squash Dhal

Rich in iron and fibre, this dhal has been made more substantial by adding butternut squash. Aubergine would be fine to use, too, or stir in handfuls of spinach at the end.

🕐 55 mins   🥧 4

- 1 tbsp rapeseed oil
- 1 onion, finely chopped
- 1 garlic clove, finely chopped
- 1 tsp each ground coriander, ground cumin and turmeric
- ½ tsp cayenne pepper (optional)
- 400g/14oz butternut squash, peeled and cut into cubes (prepared weight)
- 400g can chopped tomatoes
- 1.2 litres/2 pints vegetable stock
- 1 heaped tbsp mango chutney
- 300g/11oz red lentils
- small pack coriander, roughly chopped
- naan bread or brown rice, to serve

1 Heat the oil in a pan, add the onion and cook for 5 mins until starting to soften. Stir in the garlic and cook for a further 1 min, then stir in the spices and butternut squash.
2 Tip in the chopped tomatoes, stock and chutney and stir well. Bring to the boil, then gently simmer for about 10 mins. Add the lentils and simmer for another 20 mins until the lentils and squash are tender. Stir in the coriander and serve with warmed naan bread or brown rice.

PER SERVING 495 kcals, fat 12g, saturates 2g, carbs 58g, sugars 14g, fibre 9g, protein 42g, salt 0.6g

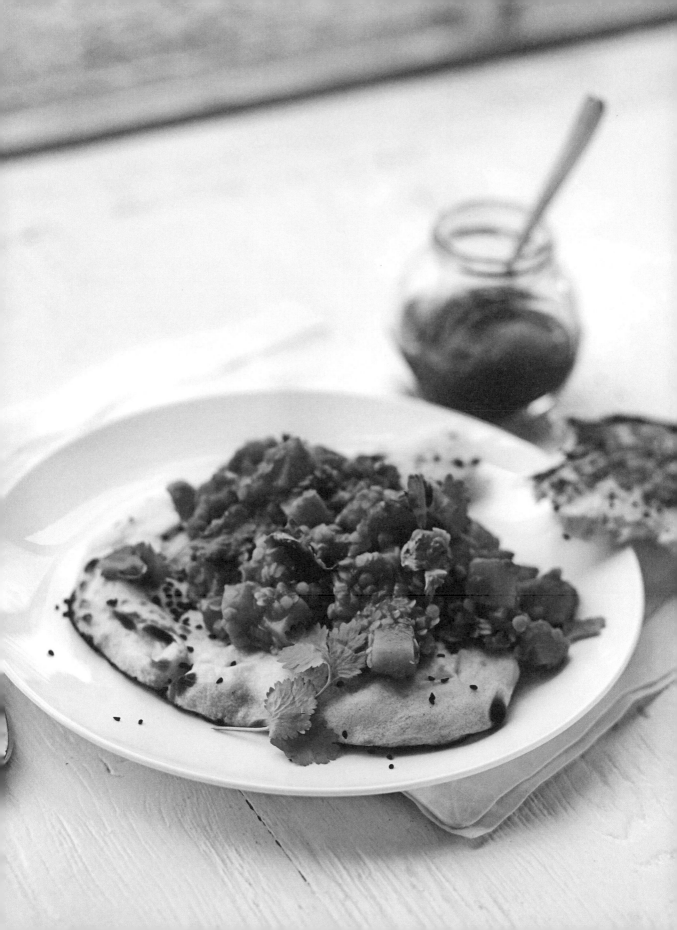

Roasted Aubergine with Bulghar & Zesty Dressing

You can use bulghar wheat or quinoa in this simple supper. Make sure the aubergine is really tender, it should be almost creamy inside.

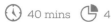 40 mins 4

- 2 aubergines, halved lengthways
- 3 tbsp olive oil
- 250g/9oz bulghar wheat
- 2 large onions, finely sliced
- 1 tbsp ground cumin
- 400g can chickpeas, drained
- handful each coriander and mint, chopped
- 1 garlic clove, crushed
- juice and zest 1 lemon

1 Heat oven to 220C/200C fan/gas 7. Score a criss-cross pattern in the cut side of the aubergines with the tip of a knife then rub all over with oil. Arrange in a roasting tin and roast for 30 mins or until the flesh is really tender.
2 Meanwhile, tip the bulghar into a pan with 1 litre of water. Bring to the boil and simmer for 15 mins until soft. Cook the onions in 2 tsp olive oil until golden and soft, add the cumin, then cook for 1 min more. Drain the bulghar and stir into the onions with the chickpeas.
3 Mix the remaining oil with the herbs, garlic and lemon zest and juice. Pile a quarter of the bulghar mix on each plate, top with half an aubergine and drizzle over some dressing.

PER SERVING 438 kcals, fat 11g, saturates 2g, carbs 71g, sugars 10g, fibre 7g, protein 14g, salt 0.38g

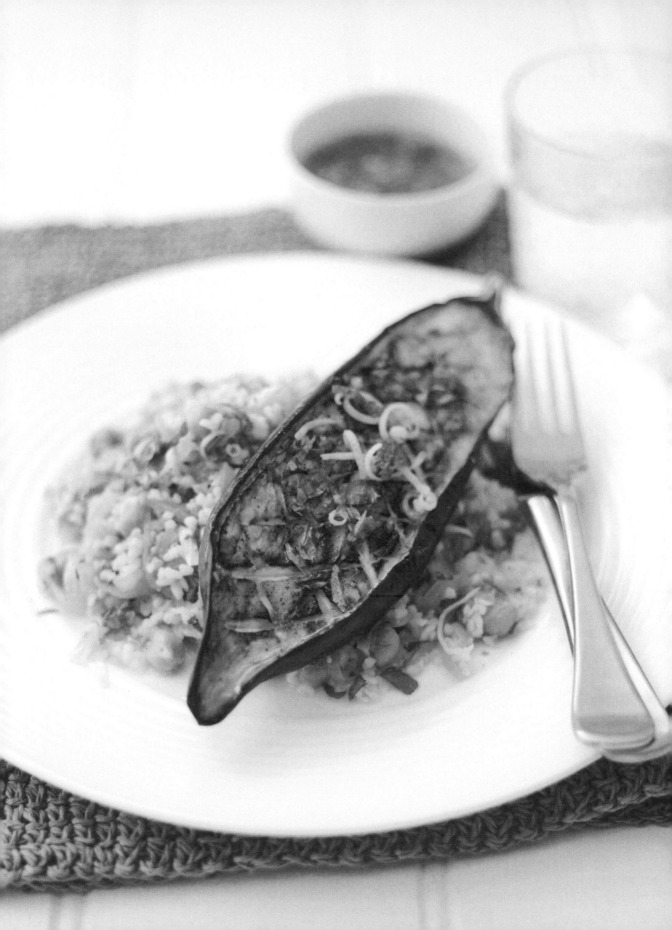

Parsnip, Rosemary & Hazelnut Risotto

Fresh herbs can be quite expensive, so if you have a garden, or just a window box, it is well worth growing a selection of woody herbs like rosemary and thyme for recipes like this.

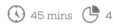 45 mins 4

- 500g/1lb 2oz parsnips, peeled, cored if large and diced
- 2 tbsp olive oil
- 1 tbsp maple syrup (optional)
- 2 rosemary sprigs, leaves finely chopped
- 2 litres/3½ pints vegetable stock
- 1 onion, finely chopped
- 2 garlic cloves, crushed
- 350g/12oz arborio risotto rice
- 25g/1oz Parmesan (or vegetarian alternative), finely grated, plus extra to serve

TO SERVE
- 25g/1oz hazelnuts, toasted and roughly chopped
- small pack flat-leaf parsley, finely chopped

1 Heat oven to 200C/180C fan/gas 6. Toss the parsnip cubes with 1 tbsp olive oil, the maple syrup, if using, and half the chopped rosemary. Spread out on a large non-stick baking sheet and roast in the oven for 20–25 mins until golden and caramelised. Heat the stock in a large saucepan and keep simmering gently.

2 Heat the remaining oil in a shallow saucepan. Add the onion, garlic and the rest of the rosemary, and cook on a low-medium heat for 5 mins until softened but not coloured. Tip in the rice and cook for 1–2 mins until hot. Add a ladleful of stock and stir constantly. Continue to add the stock gradually until the rice is cooked, about 18 mins.

3 When the rice is nearly cooked, stir in the parsnips. Take off the heat, add another splash of stock and stir in the Parmesan. Cover and leave for 2 mins, then serve with the nuts and parsley sprinkled over, and with extra Parmesan, if you like.

PER SERVING 511 kcals, fat 9g, saturates 1g, carbs 92g, sugars 16g, fibre 11g, protein 10g, salt 1.3g

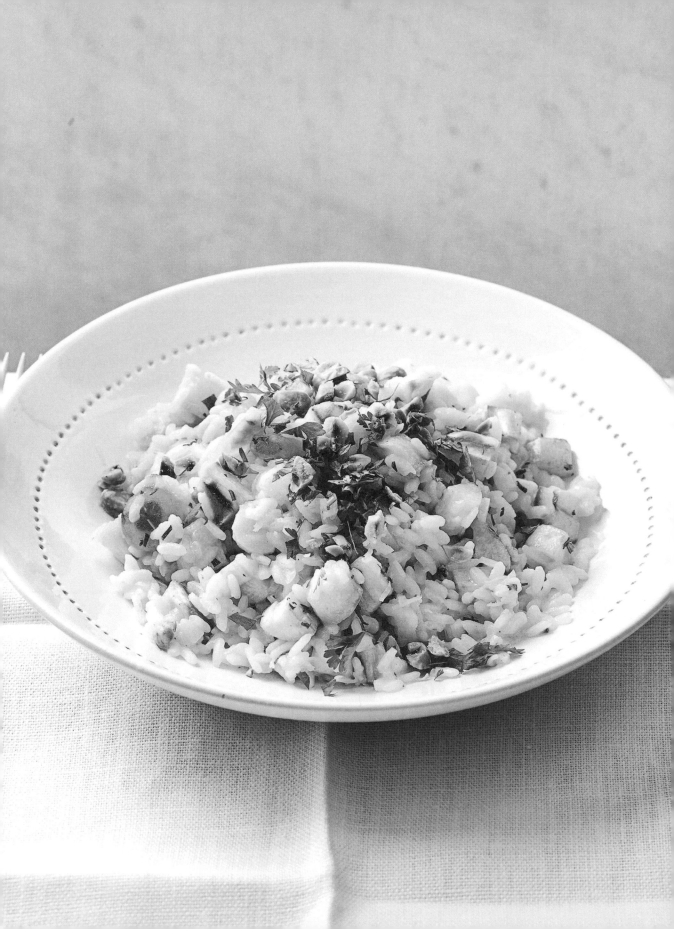

Butternut Squash Pilaf

This recipes uses a pack of fruit and nut mix, usually a blend of raisins, almonds and peanuts, but chopped dried apricots, cranberries, walnuts and hazelnuts will also work well.

🕐 40 mins 🥧 4

- 1 tbsp rapeseed oil
- 1 onion, chopped
- 1 tbsp harissa
- ½ tsp ground cinnamon
- 350g/12oz diced butternut squash (peeled weight)
- 225g/8oz brown basmati rice
- 2.5cm/1in piece root ginger, peeled and finely grated
- 1 garlic clove, crushed
- 100g/4oz fruit and nut mix
- 600ml/1 pint vegetable stock
- 1 tbsp ready-made crispy onions (optional)
- chopped parsley, to serve (optional)

1 Place a large pan over a medium heat. Add the oil and onion and cook gently until softened, around 5 mins. Tip in the harissa, cinnamon, butternut squash and rice and fry until everything is sizzling and coated in the spices. Add the ginger and garlic, fry for 30 secs more, then scatter in the fruit and nut mix. Stir in the stock and put the lid on the pan. Keep covered but stir regularly for 25-30 mins.
2 Once the rice is tender and the stock has been absorbed, serve at once on a large platter topped with crispy fried onions and chopped parsley, if you like.

PER SERVING 417 kcals, fat 13g, saturates 1g, carbs 63g, sugars 13g, fibre 5g, protein 10g, salt 0.4g

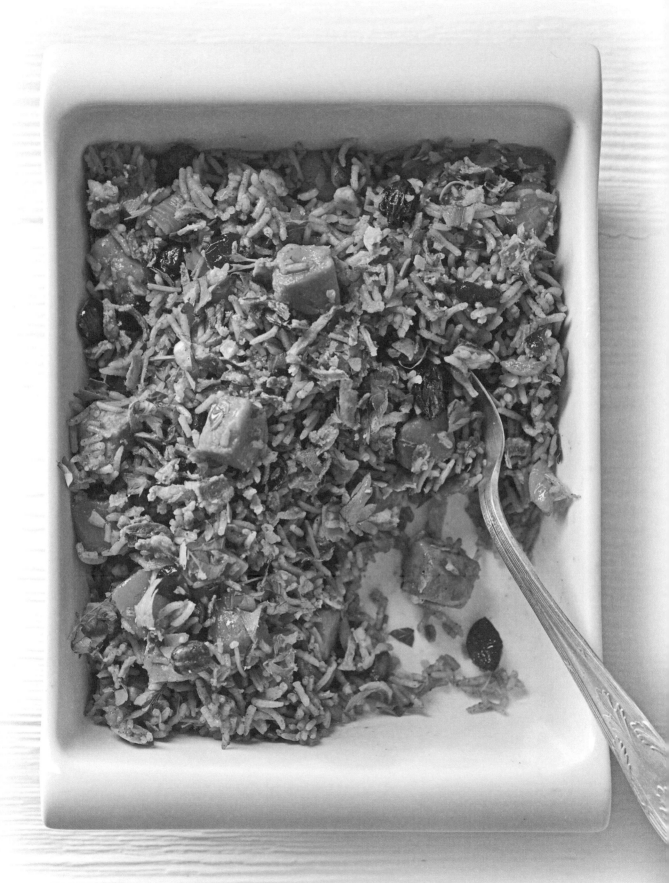

Easy Peasy Risotto with Chilli & Mint Crumbs

If you have some leftover chillies in the fridge, freeze them ready to grate into the topping of this tasty low-fat risotto.

🕐 50 mins   🥧 2-3

- 1 tbsp olive oil, plus a drizzle
- 1 onion, chopped
- 3 garlic cloves, crushed
- 200g/7oz risotto rice
- 1litre/1¾ pints vegetable stock
- 300g/11oz frozen peas
- 25g/1oz Italian-style hard cheese (pecorino, Parmesan or vegetarian alternative), grated
- juice and zest 1 lemon
- 2 slices leftover bread (a few days old is best)
- 2 frozen red chilli (deseeded if you don't like it too hot)
- ½ small bunch mint, chopped

1 Heat the oil in a large pan. Add the onion and cook for 5 mins, then add the garlic. Stir in the rice for 1–2 mins, then add the stock, a little at a time, stirring continuously until the rice is nearly cooked and the stock has all been absorbed – this will take about 20 mins. Meanwhile, tip the peas into a colander and run under the hot water tap until defrosted. Drain well, tip into a bowl and roughly mash with a potato masher.

2 Remove the risotto from the heat and stir in the peas, cheese and a squeeze of lemon juice.

3 Grate the bread on a box grater into chunky crumbs. On the finer side of the grater, grate the chilli. Heat a drizzle of oil in a frying pan, add the chilli, lemon zest and crumbs and cook for 2 mins until crispy, then add the mint and sprinkle over the risotto before serving.

PER SERVING (3) 498 kcals, fat 9g, saturates 2g, carbs 72g, sugars 7g, fibre 11g, protein 26g, salt 1.2g

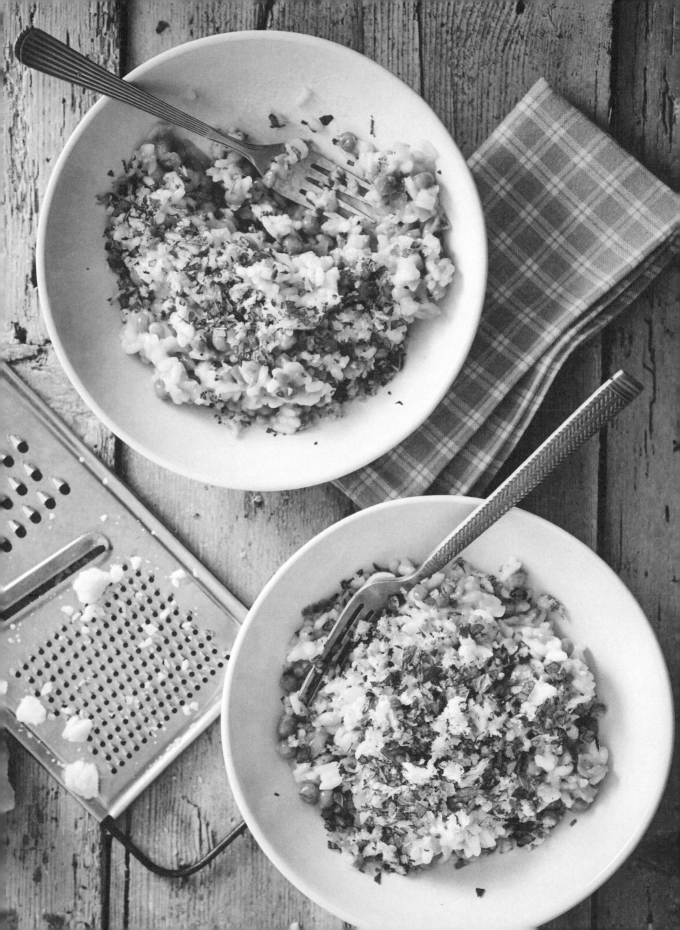

Superhealthy Pizza

Homemade pizza is easier to make than you think and needn't be loaded with fat. The portions are quite generous, so any leftovers can be enjoyed cold for lunch the next day.

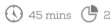 45 mins   2

- 100g/4oz each strong white and wholewheat flour
- 7g sachet fast-action dried yeast
- 125ml/4fl oz warm water

FOR THE TOPPING

- 200g can chopped tomatoes, juice drained
- handful cherry tomatoes, halved
- 1 large courgette, thinly sliced using a peeler
- 25g/1oz mozzarella, torn into pieces
- 1 tsp capers
- 8 pitted olives, roughly chopped
- 1 garlic clove, finely chopped
- 1 tbsp olive oil
- 2 tbsp chopped parsley (optional)

1 Mix the flours and yeast in a bowl, pour in the water and mix to a soft dough. Tip out onto a very lightly floured surface and knead for 5 mins until smooth and elastic. Press or roll out to a round about 30cm across then lift onto an oiled baking sheet.

2 Spread the canned tomatoes over the dough to within 2cm of the edges. Arrange the cherry tomatoes and courgette over the top, then scatter with the mozzarella. Scatter the capers, olives and garlic over the top and drizzle evenly with the oil. Cover lightly with cling film and leave to rise for 20 mins in a warm place.

3 Heat oven to 240C/220C fan/gas 9 or the highest setting then bake the pizza for 10–12 mins until crisp and golden around the edges. Scatter with the parsley, if using, and serve in wedges with salad.

PER SERVING 479 kcals, fat 13g, saturates 3g, carbs 78g, sugars 9g, fibre 10g, protein 19g, salt 1.4g

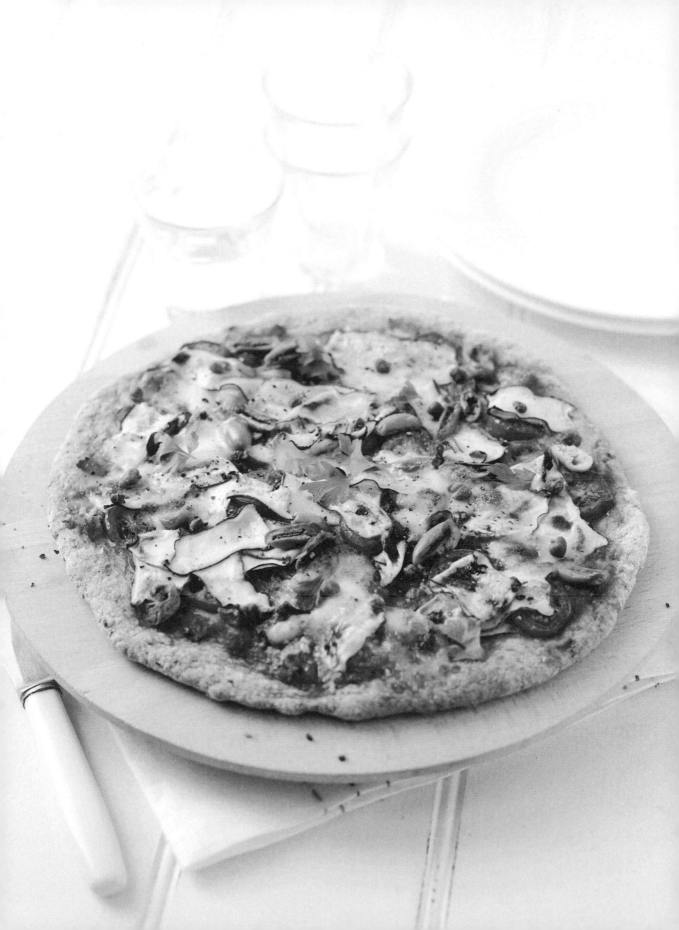

Smoky Tofu Tortillas

Made from soya beans, tofu is a good source of protein, iron, calcium, manganese, selenium, phosphorous, copper, zinc and vitamin B1. This recipe packs in 4 of your 5 a day.

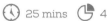 25 mins 4

- 1 tbsp rapeseed oil
- 2 onions, each cut into 12 wedges
- 2 red peppers, deseeded and sliced
- small pack coriander, leaves picked and stems finely chopped
- 2 tsp ground cumin
- 1 tsp smoked paprika
- 200g pack smoked tofu, cut into bite-sized pieces
- 400g can kidney beans, drained
- 400g can cherry tomatoes
- 1 tbsp brown sugar or maple syrup

TO SERVE
- 8 corn and wheat tortillas
- 2 limes, cut into wedges
- olive oil, for drizzling
- 1 large ripe avocado, halved, stoned, peeled and sliced just before serving
- thick yogurt

1 Heat the oil in a large frying pan and add the onions and peppers. Cook on a high heat for 8 mins or until just tender and starting to char. Add the coriander stems, fry for 1 min, stirring, then add the spices and cook for 2 mins more, stirring, until fragrant.

2 Tip in the tofu, beans, tomatoes and sugar or syrup and cook for 5 mins until the sauce is quite dry and the tofu is heated through. Warm the tortillas following the pack instructions.

3 Taste the sauce for seasoning and add the coriander leaves and a squeeze of lime. Drizzle over a little oil and serve with the tortillas, lime wedges, avocado and yogurt on the side.

PER SERVING 567 kcals, fat 16g, saturates 3g, carbs 78g, sugars 20g, fibre 15g, protein 19g, salt 1.3g

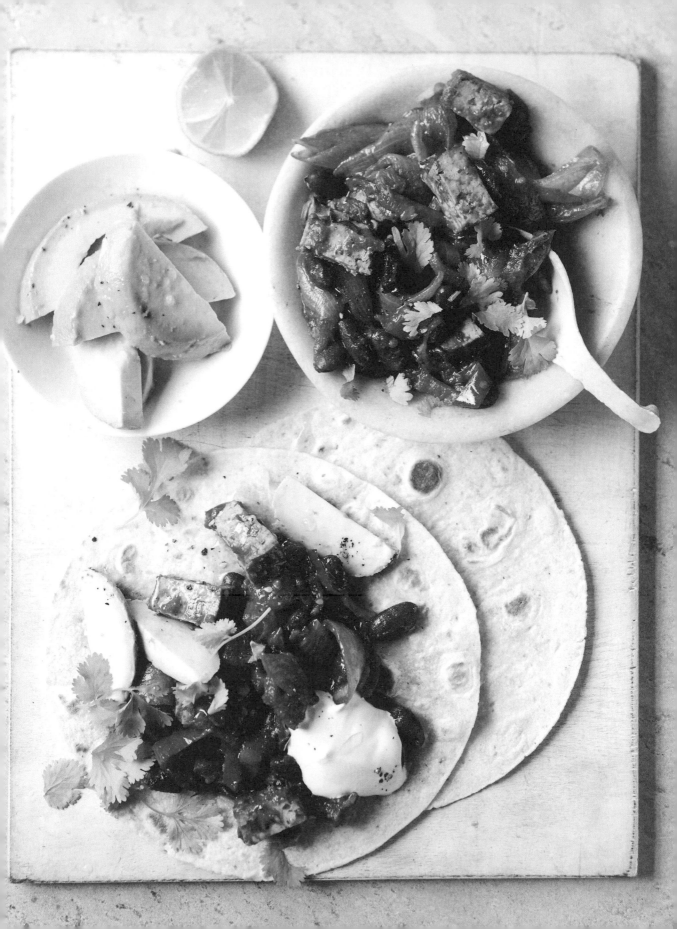

Vegetable Tagine with Chickpeas & Raisins

High in fibre and low in fat, this counts as 4 of your 5 a day. If you like your food spicy, add a dash of harissa or hot pepper sauce. Serve it with rice or wholewheat couscous.

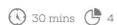 30 mins 4

- 2 tbsp olive oil
- 2 onions, chopped
- ½–1 tsp each ground cinnamon, coriander and cumin
- 2 large courgettes, cut into chunks
- 2 chopped tomatoes
- 400g can chickpeas, rinsed and drained
- 4 tbsp raisins
- 425ml/¾ pint vegetable stock
- 300g/11oz frozen peas
- chopped coriander, to serve

1 Heat the oil in a pan, then fry the onions for 5 mins until soft. Stir in the spices. Add the courgettes, tomatoes, chickpeas, raisins and stock, then bring to the boil.
2 Cover and simmer for 10 mins. Stir in the peas and cook for 5 mins more. Sprinkle with coriander to serve.

PER SERVING 264 kcals, fat 9g, saturates 1g, carbs 36g, sugars 19g, fibre 9g, protein 12g, salt 0.52g

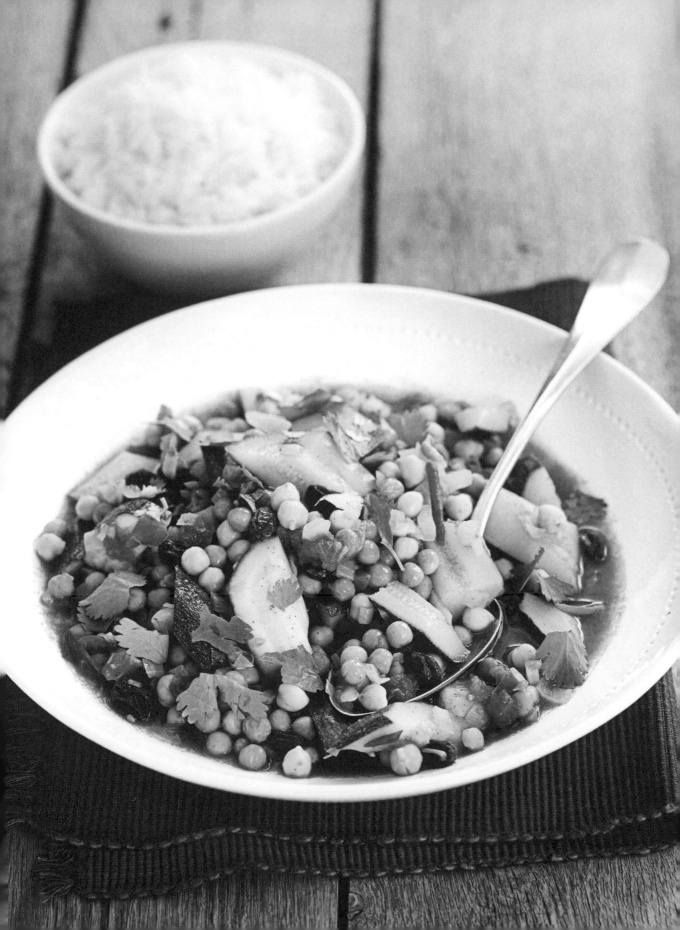

Spicy Noodles with Spring Onions & Fried Eggs

Use up leftovers from the fridge with a few store cupboard ingredients in this versatile noodle dish. If you don't have Chinese leaves try shredded cabbage, kale or blanched broccoli.

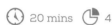 20 mins 4

- 4 nests of wholewheat noodles
- 6 spring onions, 1 very finely chopped, 5 sliced
- 1 red chilli, deseeded and finely chopped
- 2 tbsp rapeseed oil
- 1 heaped tbsp Madras curry paste
- 2 carrots, cut into discs on the diagonal then sliced
- 1 Chinese leaf cabbage, sliced
- 1 tbsp soy sauce, plus extra to taste
- 4 eggs

1 Cook the noodles following the pack instructions, meanwhile mix the chopped onions and chilli and set aside.

2 Heat half the oil in a wok, add the curry paste and cook for a couple of mins. Tip in the carrots and cook for 2 mins more. Add the sliced spring onions and cabbage and stir-fry until soft. Drain the noodles and toss into the wok with the soy sauce. Cook over the heat to warm through.

3 While the noodles are warming, heat the remaining oil in a frying pan, crack in the eggs and sprinkle the whites with the chilli mixture. Serve on the noodles with extra soy, if you like, but be sparing as it is high in salt.

PER SERVING 471 kcals, fat 16g, saturates 3g, carbs 59g, sugars 6g, fibre 6g, protein 18g, salt 2.6g

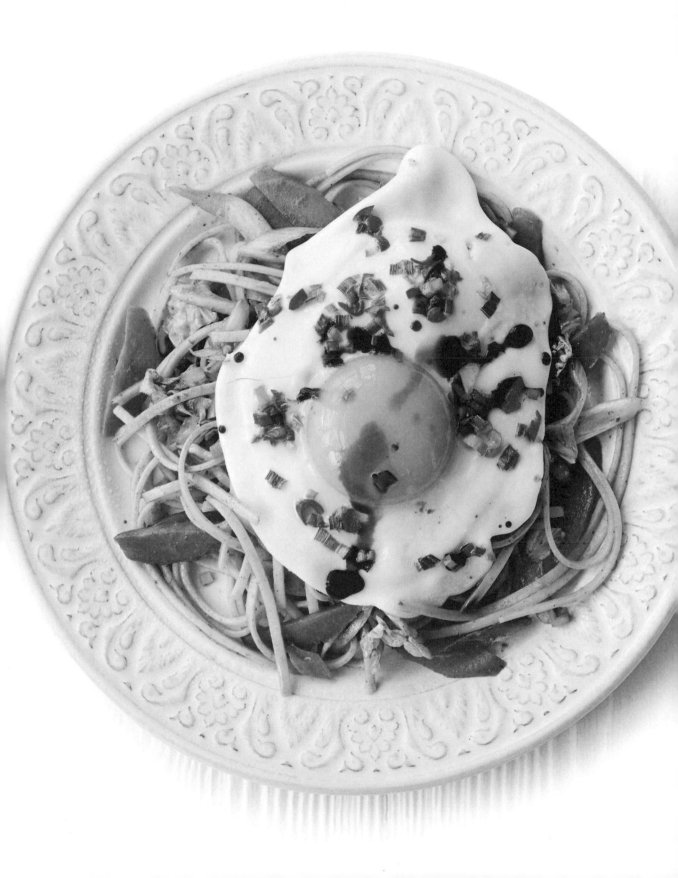

Lentil Kofta with Orzo & Feta

Canned green lentils make a good, speedy base for these koftas, but make sure you drain them really well.

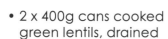 55 mins 4

- 2 x 400g cans cooked green lentils, drained
- 1 medium egg
- 100g/4oz oats
- 1 tbsp harissa
- ½ tsp each ground cumin and coriander
- small bunch parsley, chopped
- zest 1 lemon
- 2 tbsp rapeseed oil
- 4 garlic cloves, crushed
- 2 x 400g cans chopped tomatoes
- 300g/11oz orzo pasta
- 100g/4oz feta, crumbled

1 Put the lentils, egg, oats, harissa, spices, half the parsley and the lemon zest in a food processor and blitz until finely chopped. Remove the blade, shape the mixture into balls the size of cherry tomatoes, then chill for 20 mins. Heat oven to 200C/180C fan/gas 6.

2 Meanwhile, heat 1 tbsp of the oil in a pan. Add the garlic, sizzle for 30 secs, then add the tomatoes. Bubble the sauce for 20–25 mins until rich and thickened. While the sauce cooks, line a baking tray with foil and arrange the kofta on top. Drizzle over the remaining oil and bake for 20 mins, rolling around in the tray halfway through cooking. Once cooked, add the kofta to the tomato sauce, gently coating each one.

3 Cook the orzo following the pack instructions, then drain and divide between 4 plates. Top with the sauce and kofta, crumble over the feta and sprinkle with the remaining parsley.

PER SERVING 598 kcals, fat 16g, saturates 5g, carbs 82g, sugars 8g, fibre 11g, protein 26g, salt 1.3g

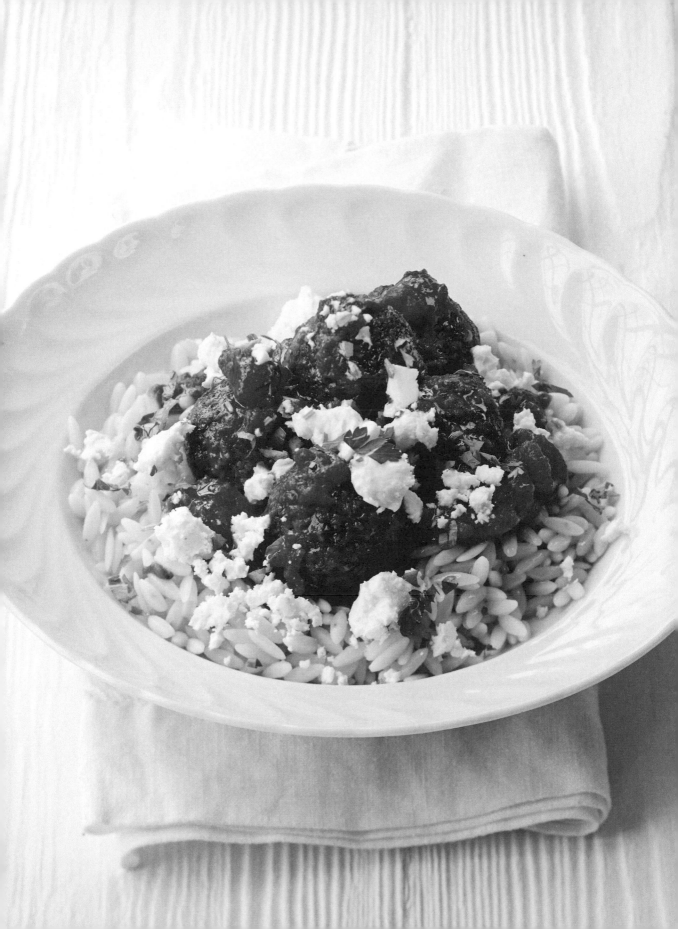

Roast Veggie Lasagne

This makes a fantastic summer supper to serve with a handful of salad leaves. If you use fresh lasagne you don't need to pre-cook it.

🕐 1 hour 15 mins   🍴 4

- 2 tbsp olive oil
- 1 onion, sliced
- 1 garlic clove, sliced
- 1 aubergine, cut into chunks
- 1 red pepper, deseeded and chopped
- 8 tomatoes, halved
- 200g/8oz lasagne sheets
- 350ml/12fl oz passata
- 6 tbsp half-fat crème fraîche
- 2 tbsp grated Parmesan

1 Heat oven to 190C/170C fan/gas 5. Toss the oil and vegetables together and roast in a large, shallow roasting tin for 35 mins or until lightly charred. Meanwhile, boil the lasagne according to pack instructions.

2 Spoon a layer of roasted veg over the bottom of a medium-size baking dish. Pour over some passata and cover with a layer of lasagne sheets. Repeat layers to use up all the roasted veg and passata, finishing with a layer of lasagne.

3 Use a spoon to dollop over the crème fraîche, then sprinkle with the Parmesan. Return to the oven for 25 mins, until the lasagne is heated through and the top is golden and bubbling.

PER SERVING 279 kcals, fat 13g, saturates 4g, carbs 35g, sugars 15g, fibre 6g, protein 9g, salt 0.63g

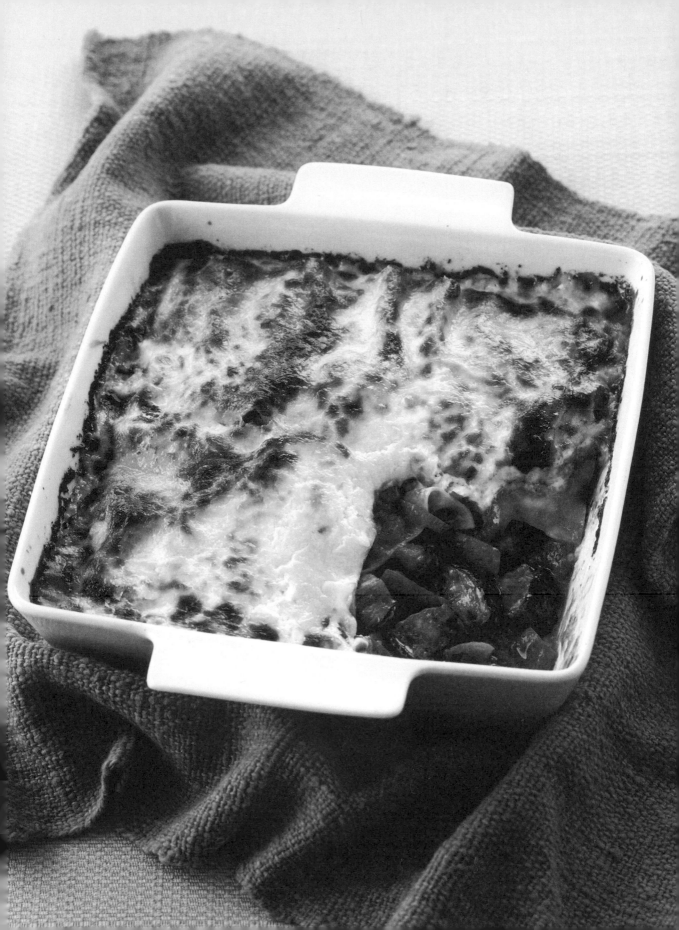

Spring Vegetable & Cauliflower Tabbouleh

Grated cauliflower makes a delicious low-carb alternative to bulghar wheat. You can use raw cauliflower here, but lightly cooking it in stock mellows the flavour and texture.

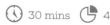 30 mins 4

- 1 whole cauliflower (about 500g/1lb 2oz when trimmed)
- 2 tbsp rapeseed oil
- 5 tbsp hot vegetable stock
- 125g pack fine asparagus, stems cut into small pieces, tips left whole
- 1 courgette, cut into small cubes
- zest 2 lemons, juice of 1
- 2 tsp sugar or maple syrup
- 2 tbsp capers, drained and chopped
- 3 tbsp olive oil
- 50g/2oz parsley, leaves only
- small pack mint, leaves only
- bunch spring onions, shredded

1 Grate the cauliflower on the coarse side of a box grater, stopping only when you get to the very hard central core. Heat 1 tbsp oil in a large pan, add the cauliflower and fry over a medium heat for 3 mins, stirring regularly. Splash in the stock, stir, then cover the pan and cook for 3–4 mins more. Stir once or twice during cooking until the cauliflower is just tender and the stock is absorbed. Spread over a plate and leave to cool. Wipe out the pan.

2 Heat the remaining rapeseed oil in the pan and add the asparagus stems and courgette. Fry over a high heat until turning golden, about 3 mins. Add the asparagus tips, fry for 2 mins more, then leave to cool.

3 Mix the lemon zest and juice, sugar or syrup, capers and olive oil to make a dressing. Chop the herbs fairly finely, then tip into a large bowl with the cauliflower, vegetables and spring onions. When ready to eat, add the dressing and mix well. Mound onto a serving plate, then cut the remaining zested lemon into wedges and serve alongside.

PER SERVING 223 kcals, fat 16g, saturates 2g, carbs 9g, sugars 7g, fibre 6g, protein 7g, salt 0.4g

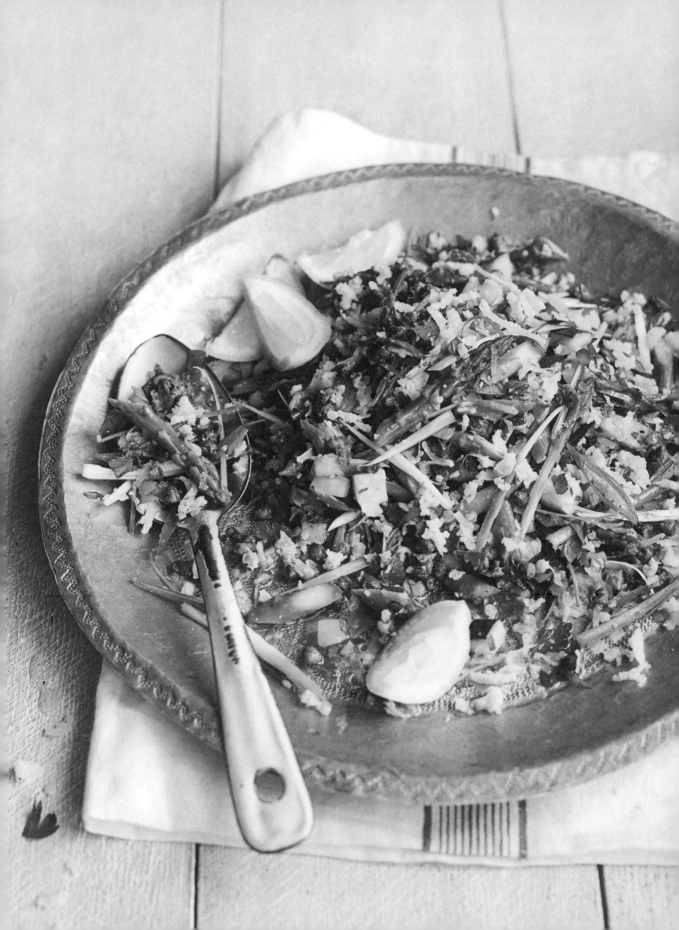

Beanballs with Tomato & Courgette Spaghetti

These are low-fat veggie alternatives to meatballs, tossed with courgette spaghetti. Using ground almonds instead of breadcrumbs increases the protein and makes them gluten-free.

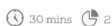 30 mins 2

- 3 garlic cloves
- 2 tsp rapeseed oil, plus extra for greasing
- 1 small onion, very finely chopped
- 2 tsp balsamic vinegar
- 100g/4oz cooked red kidney beans, canned is fine
- 1 tbsp beaten egg
- 1 tsp tomato purée
- 1 heaped tsp chilli powder
- ½ tsp ground coriander
- 15g/½oz ground almonds
- 40g/1½oz cooked fresh or frozen sweetcorn kernels
- 2 tsp soft thyme leaves or ½ tsp dried

FOR THE TOMATO NOODLES
- 2 extra large or 3 normal tomatoes, chopped
- 1 tsp tomato purée
- 1 tsp balsamic vinegar
- 2 courgettes, cut into spaghetti-like shreds with a special peeler, or cut by hand

1 Finely chop the garlic for the beanballs and sauce. Heat the oil in a large pan and fry the onions, stirring frequently for 8 mins. Stir in the balsamic vinegar and continue cooking for 2 mins more.

2 Meanwhile, put the beans in a bowl with the egg, tomato purée and spices then mash until smooth. Stir in the ground almonds and corn with the thyme, 1 chopped garlic clove and balsamic onions. Mix well and shape into about 8 balls the size of a walnut and place on a baking tray lined with oiled baking parchment.

3 Heat oven to 220C/200C fan/gas 7 and bake the meatballs for 15 mins until firm. Meanwhile, put the tomatoes, tomato purée and balsamic vinegar in a pan and cook with 2–3 tablespoons water until pulpy then stir in the remaining garlic and the courgette noodles. Turn off the heat as you want to warm the noodles rather than cook them. Serve with the beanballs.

PER SERVING 258 kcals, fat 11g, saturates 1g, carbs 24g, sugars 12g, fibre 9g, protein 12g, salt 0.7g

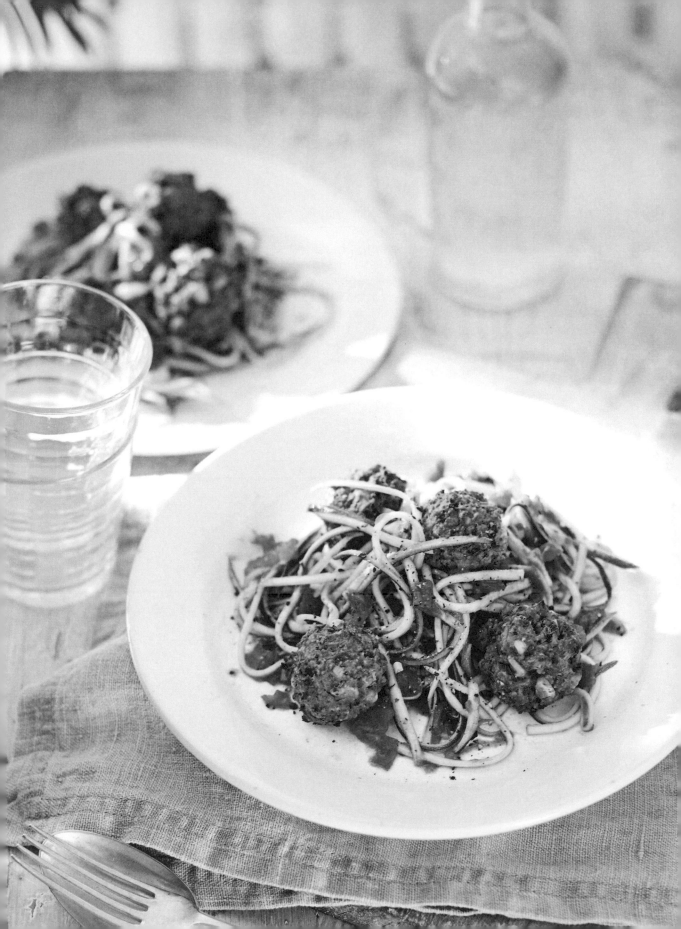

Roasted Summer Vegetable Casserole

This is low calorie, packed with vitamins and minerals and it also provides an amazing 5 of your 5-a-day!

🕐 1 hour 15 mins   🍕 2-3

- 3 tbsp olive oil
- 1 garlic bulb, halved through the middle
- 2 large courgettes, thickly sliced
- 1 large red onion, sliced
- 1 aubergine, halved and sliced on the diagonal
- 2 large tomatoes, quartered
- 200g/7oz new potatoes, scrubbed and halved
- 1 red pepper, deseeded and cut into chunky pieces
- 400g can chopped tomatoes
- ½ small pack parsley, chopped

1 Heat oven to 200C/180C fan/gas 6 and put the oil in a roasting tin. Tip in the garlic and all the fresh veg, then toss with your hands to coat in the oil and roast for 45 mins.

2 Remove the garlic from the roasting tin and squeeze out the softened cloves all over the veg, stirring to evenly distribute. In a medium pan, simmer the chopped tomatoes until bubbling, and stir through the roasted veg in the tin. Scatter over the parsley and serve.

PER SERVING (2) 474 kcals, fat 20g, saturates 3g, carbs 52g, sugars 30g, fibre 18g, protein 13g, salt 0.3g

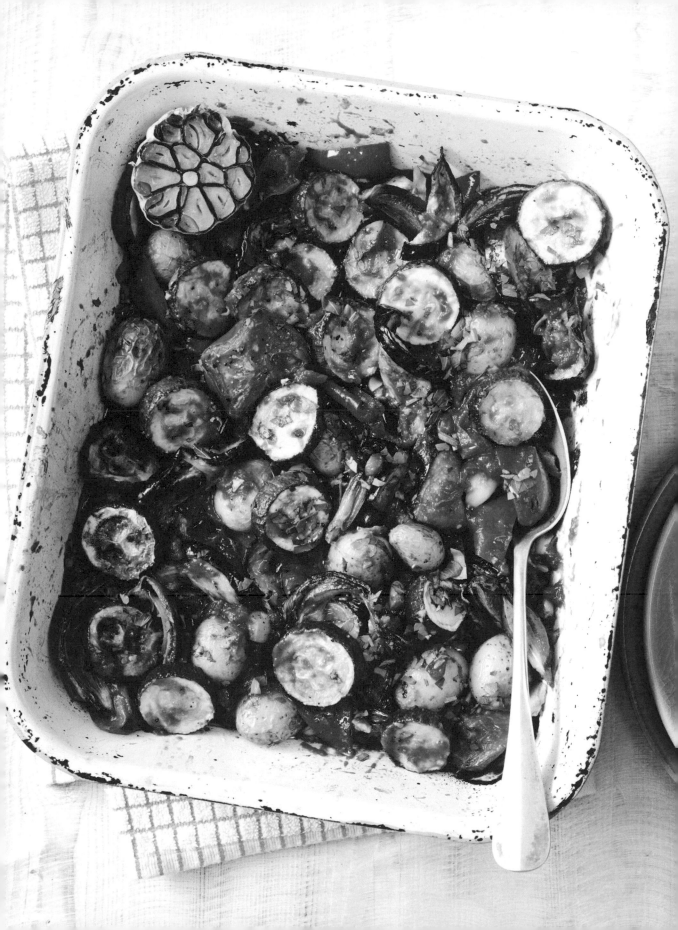

Roast Squash & Kale Salad with Orange Dressing

This tastes fresh and full of interesting flavours and textures. Eat the leftover pomegranate as a snack, scatter it over cereal for breakfast, or use it in another recipe the next day.

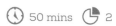 50 mins 2

- 2 red onions, each cut into 4 thick rings
- 4 garlic cloves, unpeeled
- 8 small wedges of butternut squash (prepared weight 250g/9oz)
- 2 tsp rapeseed oil
- ½ tsp caraway or fennel seeds
- ½ x 60g bag baby kale or rocket
- 50g/2oz pomegranate seeds (about ¼ of a large fruit)
- 50g/2oz feta, crumbled

FOR THE DRESSING
- 1 orange
- 1 tbsp white or red wine vinegar
- 1 tsp rapeseed oil
- 2 tbsp pumpkin seeds

1 Heat oven to 200C/180C fan/gas 6. Toss the onions, garlic and squash in the oil, then arrange in a single layer on a baking tray and roast for 25 mins.

2 Remove the garlic and set aside, turn the veg over with a fish slice, sprinkle over the caraway or fennel and return to the oven for 10 mins more.

3 To make the dressing, pare the zest from half the orange and put in a bowl. Cut the peel and pith from the orange with a sharp knife. Working over the bowl to catch the juices, cut out the segments from between the membrane. Stir in the vinegar, oil and pumpkin seeds. Discard the skin of the roasted garlic, mash the soft cloves and add to the bowl. Stir well.

4 Pile the roasted veg onto a platter or plates, top with the kale, then spoon over the dressing and toss. Scatter over the pomegranate seeds and feta, and serve.

PER SERVING 360 kcals, fat 17g, saturates 5g, carbs 24g, sugars 22g, fibre 8g, protein 13g, salt 1.0g

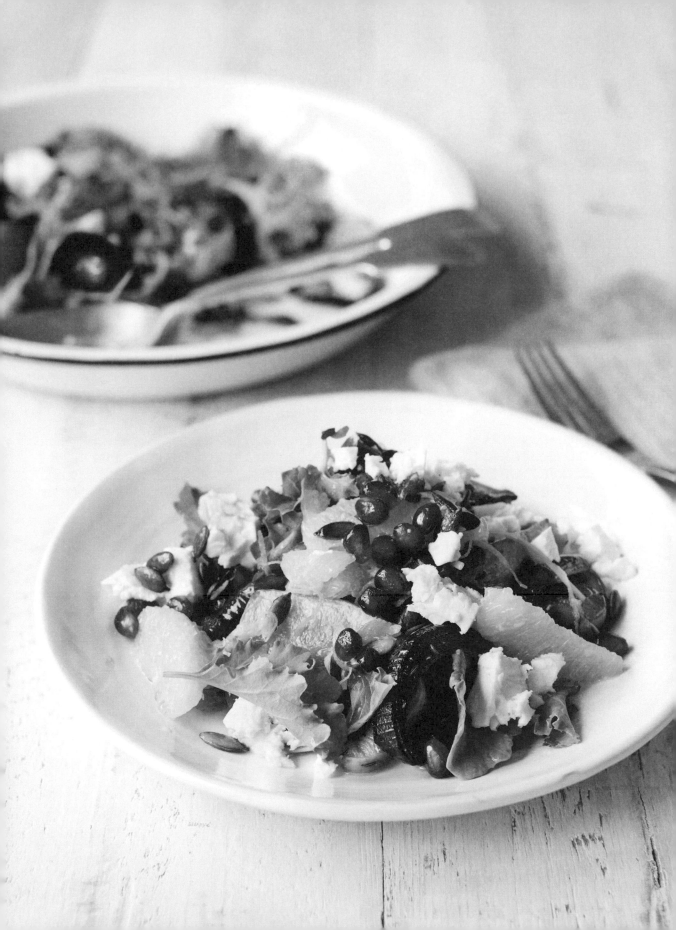

Lentil Shepherd's Pie with Celeriac & Butter Bean Mash

The traditional topping of mashed potato for a pie like this has a high GI, so this version uses mashed butter beans with celeriac for when you fancy a lighter option.

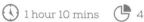 1 hour 10 mins 4

FOR THE LENTILS
- 100g/4oz red lentils
- 2 leeks, chopped
- 4 celery sticks, chopped
- 1 reduced-salt vegetable stock cube
- 150ml/5 floz red wine (or water)
- 3 heaped tbsp tomato purée
- 1 tbsp chopped thyme

FOR THE TOPPING
- 800g/1lb 12oz celeriac, peeled and chopped as though cooking potatoes
- 210g can butter beans, rinsed and drained
- 50g/2oz light soft cheese

1 Boil the celeriac with the butter beans until the celeriac is tender when tested with the point of a knife. Drain and roughly mash with the soft cheese, until the cheese is well mixed but the veg are still a little chunky.

2 Meanwhile, tip the lentils into a pan with the leeks, celery and stock cube. Pour in the red wine and 600ml water, add the tomato purée and thyme. Bring to the boil, cover the pan and simmer for 20–25 mins until the lentils are soft and pulpy. Check towards the end of cooking that they are not drying out and add a splash more water if they are.

3 Heat oven to 200C/180C fan/gas 6. Spoon the lentils into the base of four individual pie dishes then top with the celeriac mash, smoothing it to the edge of the dishes. Bake for 35 mins until bubbling and golden and serve with a green veg like broccoli.

PER SERVING 247 kcals, fat 3g, saturates 1g, carbs 26g, sugars 8g, fibre 16g, protein 14g, salt 1.2g

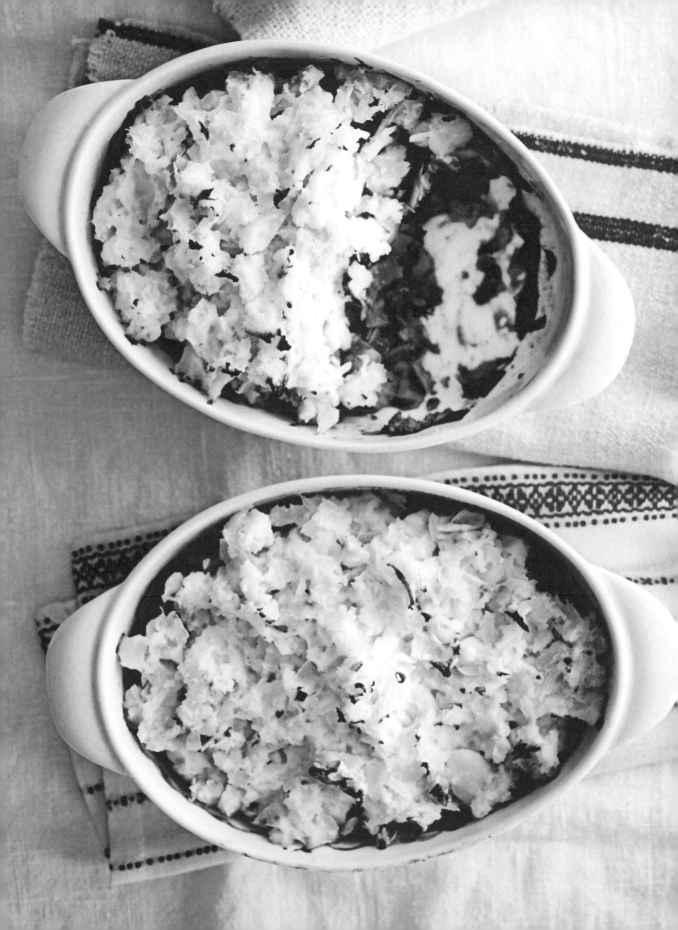

Spaghetti with Tomatoes & Basil

This is so simple yet tastes so good – although the tomatoes need to be really ripe and full flavoured – perfect if you grow your own.

🕐 15 mins   🍴 4

- 250g/9oz spaghetti, preferably wholewheat
- 2 banana shallots, finely sliced, or 1 red onion, very finely chopped
- 2 garlic cloves, finely chopped
- 4 large tomatoes, chopped
- 25 basil leaves (ideally from a growing pot)
- 100g/4oz pitted Kalamata olives
- 3 tbp olive oil
- 2 tbsp balsamic vinegar

1 Boil the pasta following the pack instructions, about 9 mins. Meanwhile, put all the remaining ingredients in a large bowl and toss together.
2 Drain the pasta well, add to the tomato mixture and toss everything together until well mixed then serve.

PER SERVING 340 kcals, fat 12g, saturates 2g, carbs 49g, sugars 6g, fibre 5g, protein 9g, salt 1.5g

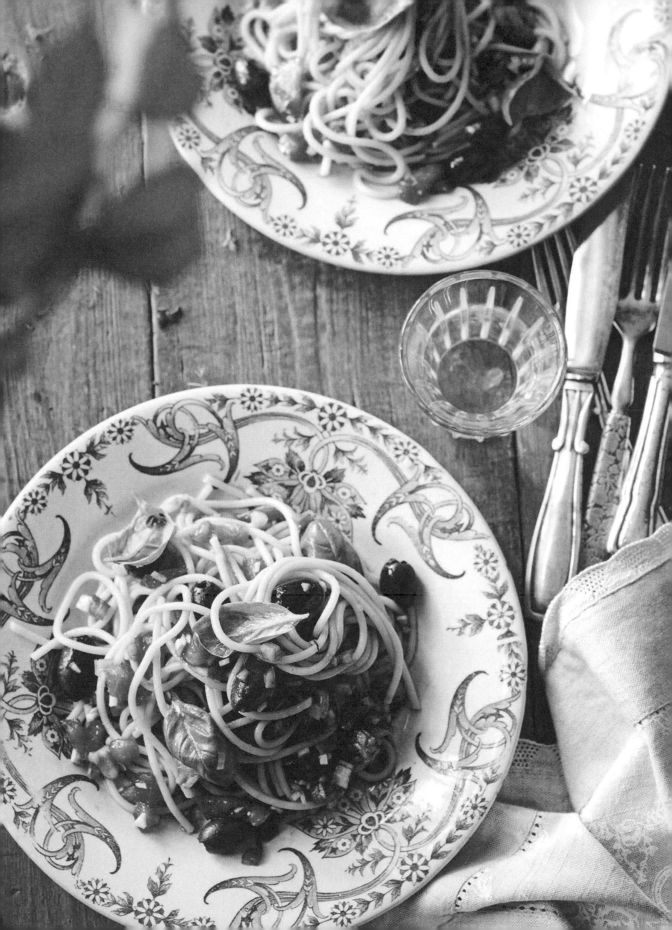

Lighter Aubergine Parmigiana

This dish tends to be loaded with oil, so our version has had a healthy makeover. If you are using dried oregano, add it with the tomatoes so it has time to impart its flavour.

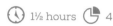 1½ hours 4

- 2 tbsp rapeseed oil, plus 1 tsp
- 2 tbsp lemon juice
- 3 aubergines (750g/1lb 10oz total weight), stalk ends trimmed, cut into 1cm/½in lengthways slices
- 1 small onion, chopped
- 3 garlic cloves, finely chopped
- 400g can and 225g can plum tomatoes
- 1 tbsp tomato purée
- 2 tbsp chopped fresh oregano or 1½ tsp dried
- 100g/4oz ricotta
- 50g/2oz mozzarella, torn into small pieces
- handful basil leaves, roughly torn
- 2 medium tomatoes, sliced
- 25g/1oz vegetarian-style Parmesan, grated

1 Heat oven to 200C/180C fan/gas 6. Measure the 2 tbsp of oil into a small bowl. Brush just a little of it onto 2 large, non-stick baking sheets (if you only have 1 tray, bake the aubergines in batches). Mix the lemon juice into the measured oil. Lay the aubergine slices snugly in a single layer on the baking sheets, brush the tops with half the oil and lemon juice, season with pepper and bake for 20 mins. Turn the slices over, give the remaining oil and lemon mixture a good stir as it will have separated, and brush it over again. Season with pepper and bake for 10–15 mins more or until softened.

2 Meanwhile, heat the remaining 1 tsp oil in a medium saucepan. Add the onion and garlic and fry for 3–4 mins, stirring often, until the onion is softened and starting to brown. Tip in both the cans of tomatoes, stir to break them up, then mix in the purée and pepper. Simmer uncovered for 10–12 mins until thickened and saucy, then stir in the oregano.

3 Spread a little of the tomato sauce in the bottom of a shallow ovenproof dish (about 25 x 20 x 5cm). Start by laying a third of the aubergine slices widthways across the dish, spread over a third of the remaining sauce and put half the ricotta on top in small spoonfuls, then half the mozzarella. Scatter over half the torn basil and season well with pepper. Repeat the layering of aubergine slices, tomato sauce, ricotta, mozzarella and basil, and finish with the final aubergine slices, the sliced tomatoes and the last of the sauce. Season with pepper and scatter over the Parmesan. Bake for about 20 mins, or until the cheese is golden and the juices are bubbling.

PER SERVING 241 kcals, fat 15g, saturates 5g, carbs 13g, sugars 11g, fibre 8g, protein 11g, salt 0.5g

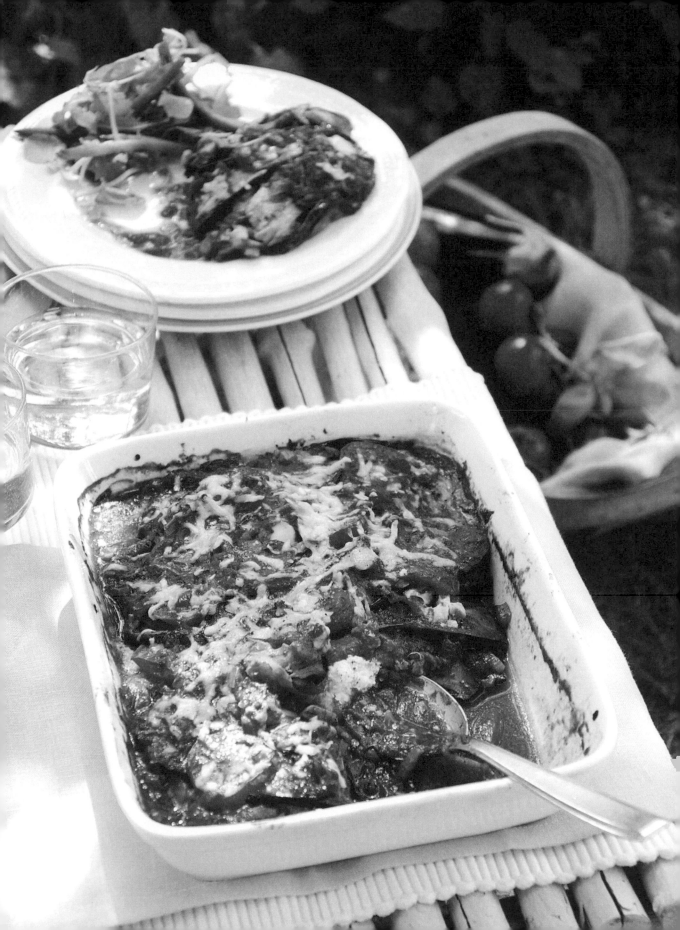

Avocado Panzanella

A mix of different-coloured tomatoes looks attractive, but it isn't essential.

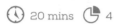 20 mins 4

- 800g/1lb 12oz mix of ripe tomatoes
- 1 garlic clove, crushed
- 1½ tbsp capers, drained and rinsed
- 1 ripe avocado, halved, stoned, peeled and chopped
- 1 small red onion, very thinly sliced
- 175g/6oz ciabatta or wholewheat crusty loaf
- 4 tbsp olive oil
- 2 tbsp red or white wine vinegar
- small handful basil leaves

1 Halve or roughly chop the tomatoes (depending on size) and put them in a bowl. Season with black pepper and add the garlic, capers, avocado and onion, and mix well. Set aside for 10 mins.

2 Meanwhile, tear or slice the ciabatta into 3cm chunks and place in a large serving bowl or on a platter. Drizzle with half the olive oil, half the vinegar and add some seasoning. When ready to serve, pour over the tomatoes and any juices. Scatter with the basil leaves and drizzle over the remaining oil and vinegar. Give it a final stir and serve immediately.

PER SERVING 332 kcals, fat 21g, saturates 4g, carbs 30g, sugars 8g, fibre 6g, protein 7g, salt 0.9g

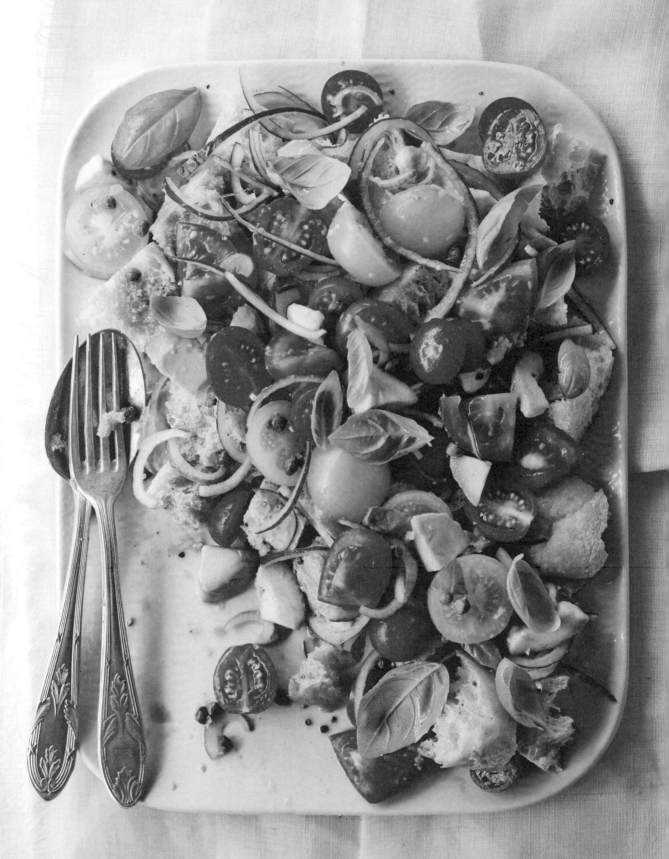

Minty Roast Veg & Houmous Salad

A layer of houmous makes a tasty base to serve a medley of roasted vegetables on top. You could also add a handful of rocket, although this already provides 4 or your 5 a day!

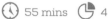 55 mins 4

- 4 parsnips, peeled and cut into wedges
- 4 carrots, cut into wedges
- 2 tsp cumin seeds
- 400g can chickpeas, drained
- 2 tbsp rapeseed oil
- 500g pack cooked beetroot (not in vinegar), drained and cut into wedges
- 2 tbsp clear honey or maple syrup
- 200g pot houmous
- 2 tbsp white or red wine vinegar
- small bunch mint, leaves picked
- 200g block Greek-style salad cheese

1 Heat oven to 200C/180C fan/gas 6. Toss the parsnips, carrots, cumin seeds and chickpeas with the oil and some seasoning in a large roasting tin. Cook for 30 mins, tossing halfway through cooking.
2 Add the beetroot to the tin and drizzle over the honey or maple syrup, then return to the oven for 10 mins. Spread the houmous thinly over a large platter, or divide between 4 dinner plates. When the veg is ready, drizzle with the vinegar and toss together in the tin. Tip the roasted vegetables on top of the houmous, scatter over the mint and cheese, drizzle with any juices from the tin and serve.

PER SERVING 611 kcals, fat 26g, saturates 9g, carbs 61g, sugars 36g, fibre 20g, protein 23g, salt 3.5g

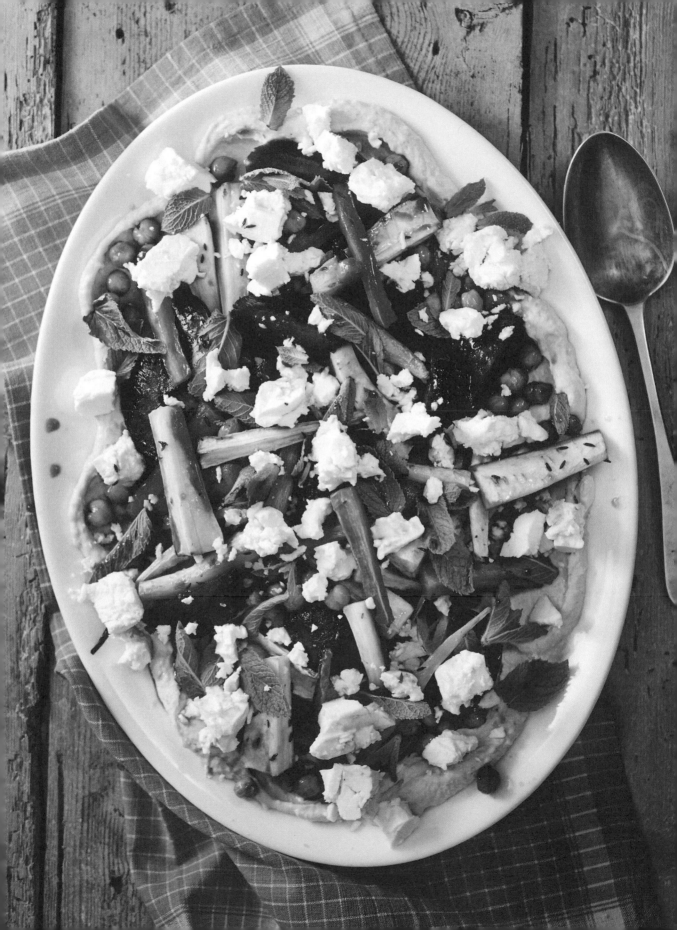

Spinach & Sweet Potato Tortilla

This unusual tortilla uses sweet potato, which unlike normal potatoes contributes towards your 5 a day. Any leftover is delicious for lunch the next day.

🕐 1 hour 10 mins   🥧 6-8

- 300g bag baby spinach leaves
- 8 tbsp olive oil
- 2 large onions, thinly sliced
- 4 medium sweet potatoes (800g/1lb 12oz), peeled and cut into thin slices
- 2 garlic cloves, finely chopped
- 8 large eggs

1 Put the spinach in a large colander and pour over a kettleful of boiling water. Drain well and, when cooled a little, squeeze dry, trying not to mush up the spinach too much.

2 Heat 3 tbsp oil in a 25cm non-stick pan with a lid, then sweat the onions for 15 mins until really soft but not coloured. Add another 3 tbsp oil and add the potatoes and garlic. Mix in with the onions, season well, cover and cook over a gentle heat for another 15 mins or so until the potatoes are very tender. Stir occasionally to stop them catching.

3 Whisk the eggs in a large bowl, tip in the cooked potato and onion, and mix together. Separate the spinach clumps, add to the mix and fold through, trying not to break up the potato too much.

4 Add 2 tbsp more oil to the pan and pour in the sweet potato and egg mix. Cover and cook over a low-medium heat for 20 mins until the base and sides are golden brown and the centre has mostly set. Run a palette knife around the sides to stop it from sticking.

5 To turn the tortilla over, put a plate face down onto the pan, then flip it over. Slide the tortilla back into the pan and cook for a further 5–10 mins until just set and golden all over. (Don't worry if it breaks up a little on the edges as you're turning it – it will look perfect when it's cooked through and set.) Continue cooking on the other side until just set and golden all over. Again, use a palette knife to release the tortilla from the sides. Allow to rest for 5 mins, then tip onto a board before cutting into wedges.

PER SERVING (8) 306 kcals, fat 17g, saturates 3g, carbs 26g, sugars 9g, fibre 5g, protein 9g, salt 0.4g

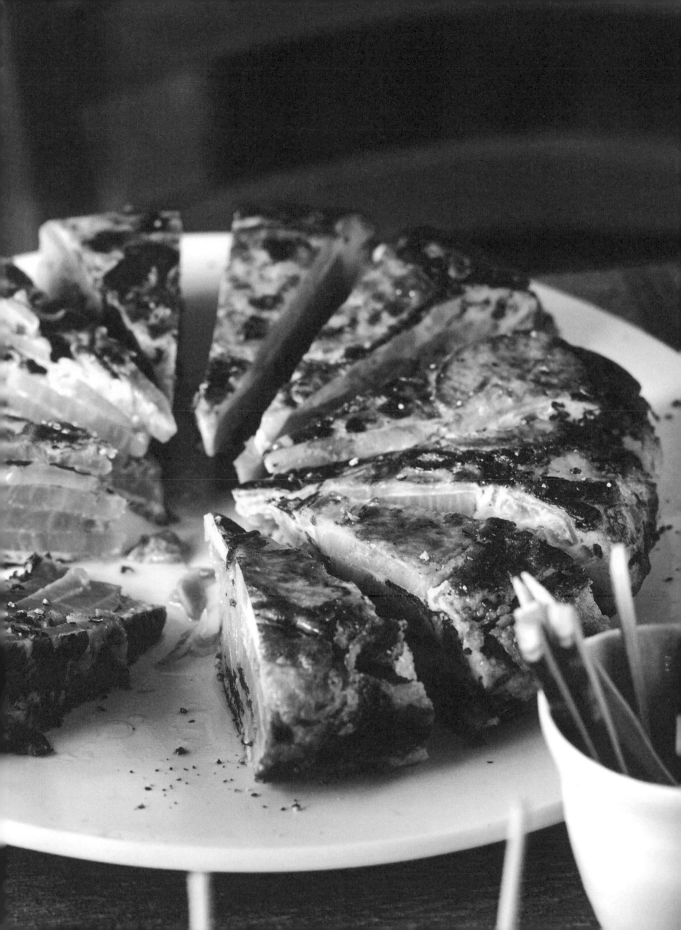

Courgette Tortilla Wedges with Pesto & Rocket

Eggs are an excellent source of protein and as a tortilla make a substantial supper. This version uses courgettes instead of potatoes, to keep the carbs low, sandwiched with pesto.

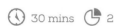 30 mins 2

- 4 tsp olive oil
- 2 courgettes (about 300g/11oz), sliced into rounds about the thickness of a £1 coin
- 6 large eggs
- 1 large garlic clove, finely grated
- 10 cherry tomatoes (or 2 clusters of 5 on the vine)
- 3 tbsp pesto, preferably fresh
- handful rocket

1 Heat 2 tsp olive oil in a non-stick frying pan about 25cm across, add the courgette slices and cook for 5 mins, until softened, stirring occasionally. Meanwhile, beat the eggs with seasoning and the grated garlic in a large bowl.

2 Tip the courgettes from the pan and wipe it out with kitchen paper. Add the remaining oil to the pan and return to the heat. Stir the courgettes into the eggs then pour into the frying pan and cook over a low heat for 10 mins until almost completely set. Slide onto a large plate then flip back into the pan and briefly cook the other side to set the last bit of raw egg. If you are nervous about flipping it over you can grill the top instead. Remove from the pan onto a board and add the tomatoes to the pan – soften a little for 2–3 mins and char the skins. Cut the tortilla in half and spread one half with 2 tbsp of the pesto and top with the other one. Cut into wedges and top each with the remaining pesto, tomatoes and rocket.

PER SERVING 450 kcals, fat 35g, saturates 7g, carbs 8g, sugars 6g, fibre 4g, protein 24g, salt 2.2g

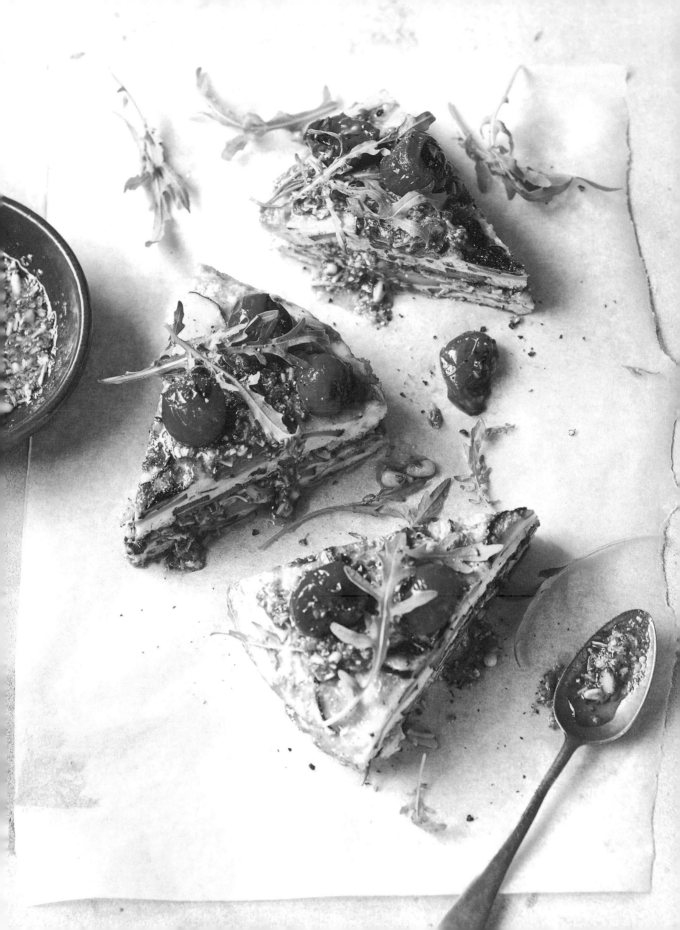

Bean Salad with Yogurt Avocado Dressing

Frozen broad beans are a great freezer standby for padding out salads, but some people find their casing a little leathery. If so, try frozen soy beans instead as they are more tender.

🕐 30 mins 🥧 4

- 2 round wholemeal pitta breads, split in half and cut into triangles
- 200g/7oz frozen baby broad beans
- 1 avocado, peeled, stoned and flesh scooped out
- 8 tbsp low-fat natural yogurt
- 1 garlic clove, roughly chopped
- 1 lemon, zest of ½, juice of whole
- 2 Little Gem lettuces, roughly chopped
- 400g can cannellini beans, rinsed and drained
- 4 spring onions, finely chopped
- 2 carrots, peeled and grated
- 10 radishes, halved
- handful of snipped cress

1 Heat grill to high. Spread the pitta triangles out in a shallow baking tray. Toast for a couple of mins to crisp, turning once. Keep a close eye on them otherwise they will burn. Once toasted, remove and place to one side. Next, pop the broad beans in boiling water and cook for 2–3 mins, then drain. If you like you can remove the bright green bean from the hard outer shell, but it isn't essential.

2 In a blender, whizz together the avocado, yogurt, garlic, lemon juice and zest.

3 Put the remaining ingredients in a bowl, except the cress. Toss together with the avocado and yogurt dressing, then sprinkle over the pitta croutons and cress. Eat straight away.

PER SERVING 260 kcals, fat 7g, saturates 2g, carbs 38g, sugars 10g, fibre 9g, protein 12g, salt 0.7g

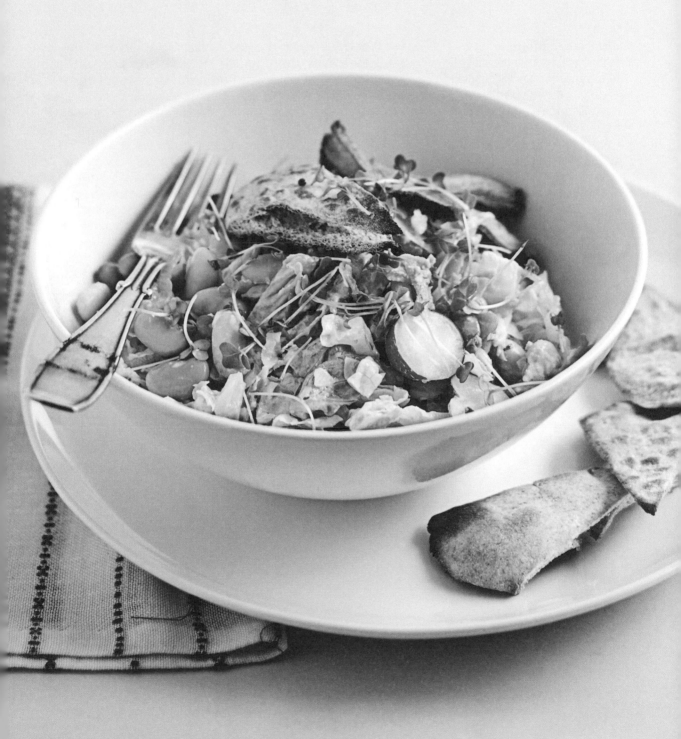

Falafel Scotch Eggs

These are fantastic for supper, but equally at home on a veggie picnic.

🕐 55 mins 🥧 8

- 9 large eggs
- 1 tbsp rapeseed oil, plus extra for rolling and frying
- 2 large onions, chopped
- 2 garlic cloves, crushed
- 1 tbsp ground cumin
- 1 tbsp ground coriander
- 400g can chickpeas, rinsed and drained
- ½ pack coriander, leaves only
- 200g/7oz wholewheat breadcrumbs
- 5 tbsp plain flour, plus extra for dusting
- 25g/1oz dried breadcrumbs
- 3 tbsp sesame seeds
- rapeseed oil, for frying

1 Put 8 of the eggs in a pan of cold water. Bring to the boil, cook for 5 mins, then quickly lift out of the pan and plunge in a big bowl of cold water to cool. Once cool enough to handle, peel.

2 While the eggs cool, put the oil, onions and garlic in a frying pan. Fry very gently until really soft and just starting to turn golden. Add the spices and fry for a few mins more. Tip into a food processor and whizz to a paste, then add the chickpeas and coriander leaves and pulse until finely chopped but not pasty. Stir in the wholemeal breadcrumbs, flour and final egg, beaten first with a fork.

3 Divide the mixture into 8. Take a portion at a time and flatten between your hands (rub your hands with a little more oil if it's sticking to your fingers too much). Roll 1 of your peeled eggs in a little flour, shake to remove the excess, then wrap the falafel mixture around it, moulding it to completely cover the egg and squishing it together at the joins to seal. Repeat to cover all the eggs. Tip the dried breadcrumbs onto a plate and mix in the sesame seeds. Roll each egg in it to coat. Can be made 1 day ahead, loosely covered with cling film and chilled.

4 Get a large, deep saucepan and half-fill it with oil, or use a deep-fat fryer. Heat until a bit of bread browns in about 30 secs. Add a couple of eggs at a time and fry, turning, until really golden and crisp, about 2 mins. Lift onto kitchen paper to drain really well while you cook the rest of the eggs in batches. Eat warm or cold, and serve with tomato chutney, if you like.

PER EGG 404 kcals, fat 26g, saturates 4g, carbs 29g, sugars 3g, fibre 5g, protein 15g, salt 0.7g

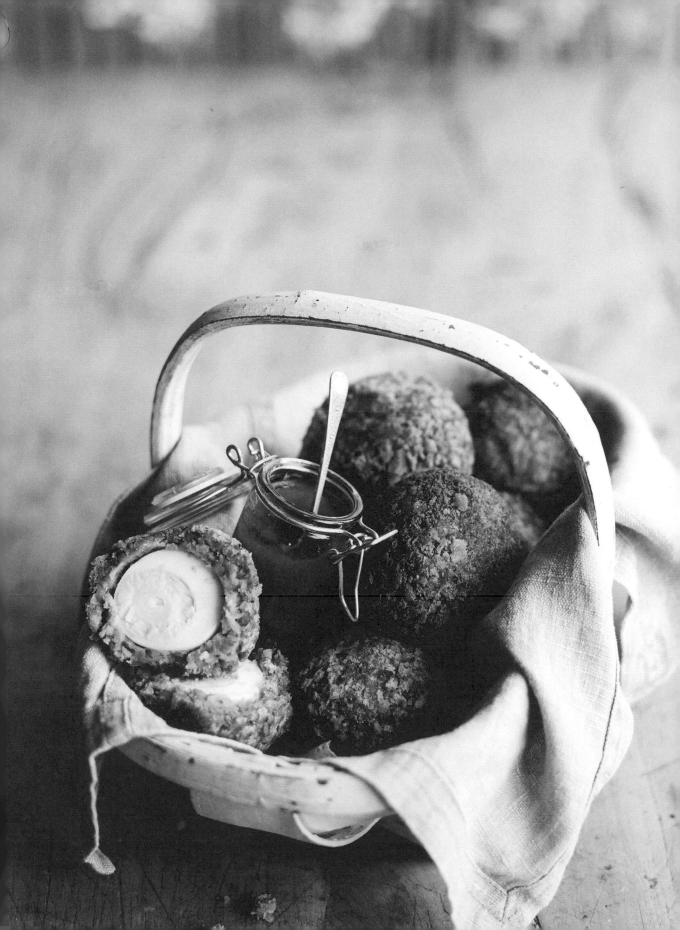

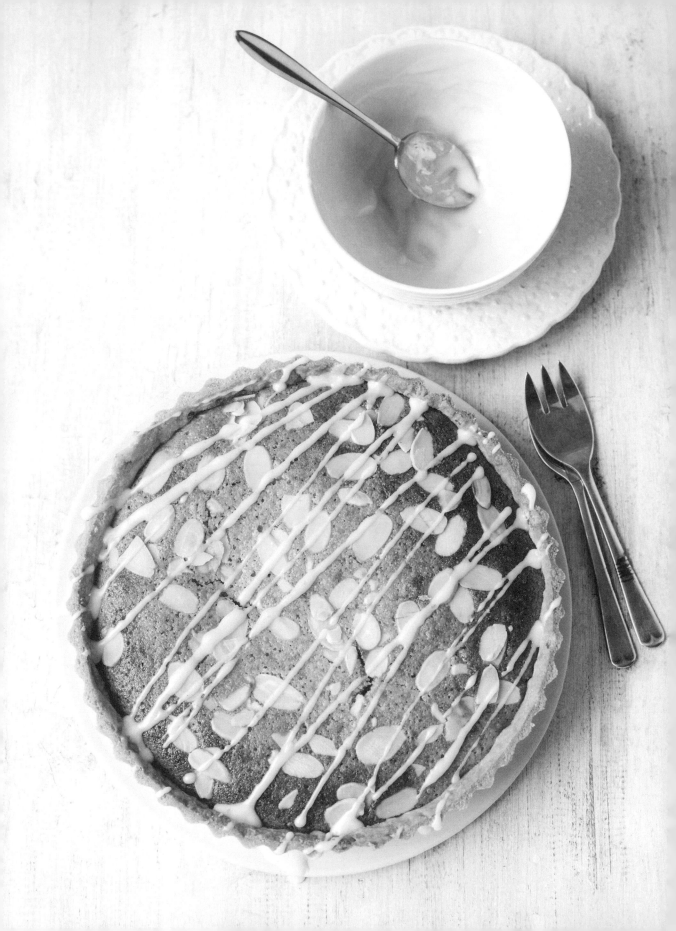

Chapter 6:

HEALTHY BREADS, LIGHTER BAKES & PUDDINGS

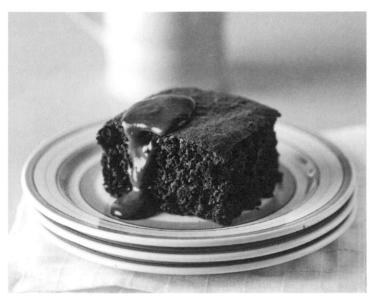
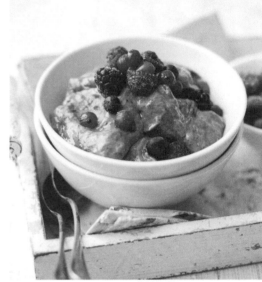
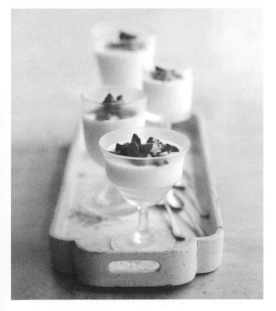
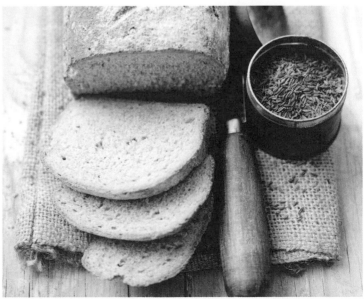

Rye Bread

This rye bread recipe is lower in gluten than most white loaves because it uses white or wholemeal flour, depending on the lightness you want. Rye keeps you feeling fuller for longer.

🕐 50 minutes, plus rising and proving ◐ Makes 1 loaf

- 200g/7oz rye flour, plus extra for dusting
- 200g/7oz strong white or wholemeal flour
- 7g sachet fast-action dried yeast
- ½ tsp salt
- 1 tbsp clear honey
- a little rapeseed oil, for greasing
- 1 tsp caraway seed (optional)

1 Tip the flours, yeast and salt into a bowl. In a jug, mix the honey with 250ml warm water, pour the liquid into the bowl and mix to form a dough. Rye flour can be quite dry and absorbs lots of water, if the dough looks too dry add more warm water until you have a soft dough. Tip out onto a lightly floured work surface and knead for 10 mins until smooth. Rye contains less gluten than white flour so the dough will not feel as springy as a conventional white loaf.

2 Place the dough in a well-oiled bowl, cover with cling film and leave to rise in a warm place for 1–2 hrs, or until roughly doubled in size. Dust a 900g/2lb loaf tin with flour.

3 Tip the dough back onto a lightly floured work surface and knead briefly to knock out any air bubbles. If using caraway seeds work these into the dough. Shape into a smooth oval loaf and pop into your tin. Cover the tin with oiled cling film and leave to rise somewhere warm for a further 1–1 hr 30 mins, or until doubled in size.

4 Heat oven to 220C/200C fan/gas 7. Remove the cling film and dust the surface of the loaf with rye flour. Slash a few incisions on an angle then bake for 30 mins until dark brown and hollow sounding when tapped. Transfer to a wire cooling rack and leave to cool for at least 20 mins before serving.

PER SERVING (8) 170 kcals, fat 1g, saturates 0.2g, carbs 34g, fibre 7g, sugars 2g, protein 6g, salt 0.3g

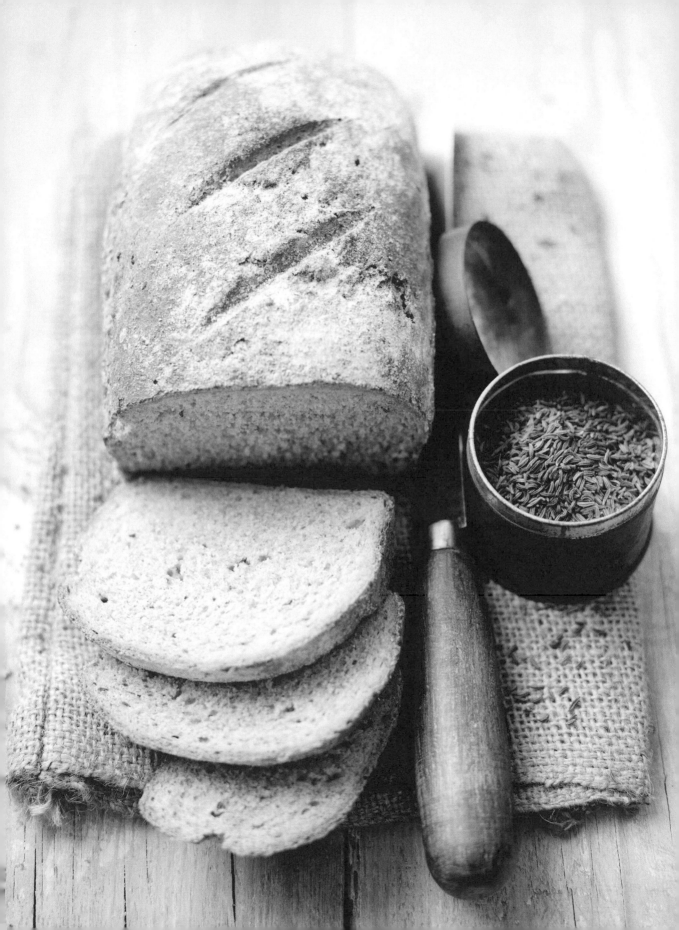

Malted Nut & Seed Loaf

Add seeds, nuts and wholemeal flour to a basic dough for a bread with bags of flavour and nutrient goodness.

🕐 1 hour, plus rising   🕐 Cuts into 12 slices

- 100g/4oz mixed seeds (we used a mix of linseeds, hemp seeds, pumpkin seeds and sesame seeds)
- 500g/1lb 2oz strong wholemeal flour
- 7g sachet fast-action yeast
- 1 tsp salt
- 50g/2oz walnut pieces
- a little sunflower oil, for greasing

1 Set aside 1 tbsp of seeds, then mix all the dry ingredients together in a large bowl and make a well in the middle. Stir in the seeds and nuts. Pour in up to 350ml/12fl oz lukewarm water and mix to a slightly wet dough.

2 Tip out on to a lightly floured surface and knead for 10 mins or until smooth and elastic. Put in a clean, oiled bowl, cover and leave until doubled in size. Roll the dough around in the reserved seeds, then lift the bread onto a tray to prove for about 30 mins until doubled in size.

3 Heat oven to 220C/200C fan/gas 7. Bake the bread for 15 mins, then lower the oven temperature to 190C/170C fan/gas 5 and continue to bake for 30 mins until the loaf sounds hollow when removed from the tin and tapped on the base. Leave on a wire rack to cool completely.

PER SLICE 172 kcals, fat 4g, saturates 1g, carbs 28g, sugars 1g, fibre 5g, protein 7g, salt 0.43g

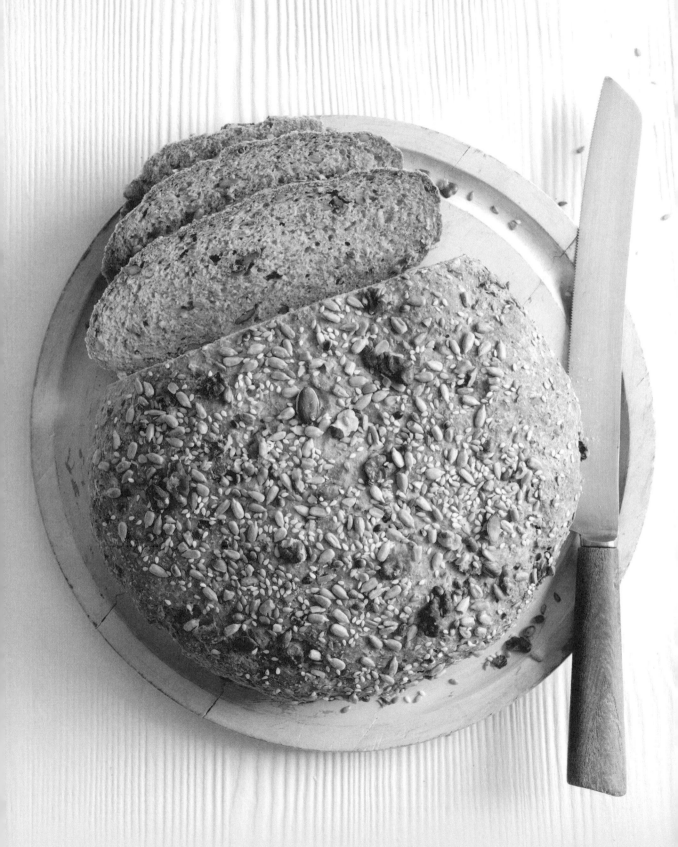

Cinnamon Cashew Flapjacks

Cinnamon can help maintain a healthy heart and normal levels of glucose and fat. It helps reduce inflammation and is said to even play a role in protecting the body from free radicals.

🕐 55 mins ◗ Makes 15

- 140g/5oz butter, plus extra for greasing
- 140g/5oz light brown soft sugar
- 2 tbsp set honey
- 1 tbsp ground cinnamon
- 140g/5oz porridge oats
- 85g/3oz desiccated coconut
- 85g/3oz sesame seeds
- 50g/2oz sunflower seeds
- 1 tbsp plain flour
- 85g/3oz cashews or pecans

1 Heat oven to 160C/140C fan/gas 3. Grease and line a 20 x 30cm cake tin with baking parchment. Melt the butter in a large non-stick pan, add the sugar, honey and cinnamon, and stir with a wooden spoon over a low heat for 5–10 mins until the sugar dissolves.

2 Remove from the heat and stir in all the remaining ingredients until well coated in the spice mixture. Tip into the tin and press down to an even layer. Bake for 30–35 mins until golden. Cool for 5 mins, then mark into squares – don't remove from the tin yet as they won't hold together until they are cold. Will keep in a sealed container for a couple of days.

PER FLAPJACK 282 kcals, fat 19g, saturates 9g, carbs 20g, sugars 12g, fibre 3g, protein 5g, salt 0.2g

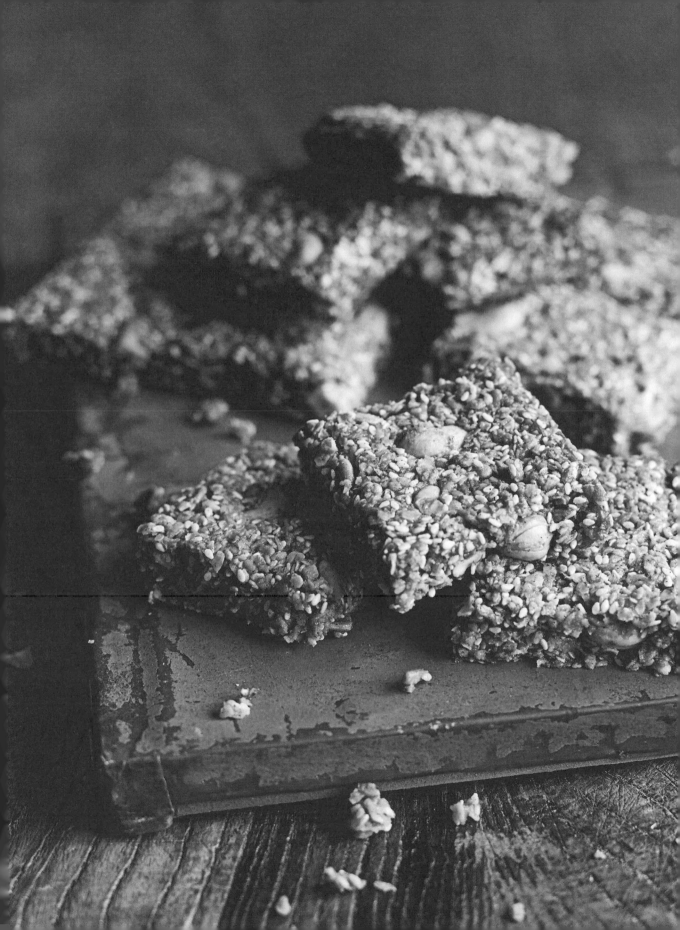

Healthy Banana Bread

Have your cake and eat it with this low-fat banana bread, perfect with a cup of tea, or even for breakfast.

🕐 1 hour 35 mins   🥧 Cuts into 10 slices

- butter or low-fat spread, for the tin, plus extra to serve
- 140g/5oz wholemeal flour
- 100g/4oz self-raising flour
- 1 tsp each bicarbonate of soda and baking powder
- 300g/11oz mashed banana, from overripe black bananas
- 4 tbsp maple syrup or honey
- 3 large eggs, beaten with a fork
- 150ml pot low-fat natural yogurt
- 25g/1oz chopped pecans or walnuts (optional)

1 Heat oven to 160C/140C fan/gas 3. Grease and line a 900g/2lb loaf tin with baking parchment (allow it to come 2cm above the top of the tin). Mix the flours, bicarb and baking powder in a large bowl.

2 Mix the bananas, syrup or honey, eggs and yogurt. Quickly stir into dry ingredients, then gently scrape into the tin and scatter with nuts, if using. Bake for 1 hr 10 mins–1 hr 15 mins or until a skewer comes out clean.

3 Cool in the tin on a wire rack. Eat warm or at room temperature, on its own or with butter or low-fat spread.

PER SLICE 132 kcals, fat 2g, saturates 1g, carbs 22g, sugars 7g, fibre 3g, protein 5g, salt 0.6g

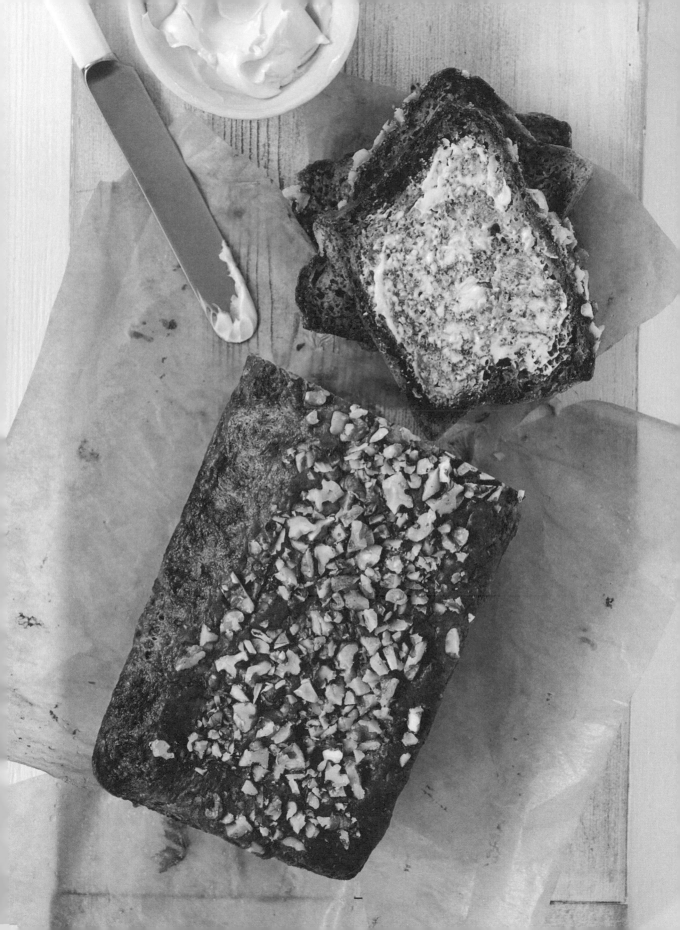

Lighter Lemon Drizzle Cake

Yogurt and omega 3-rich rapeseed oil combine to replace butter in this lower-fat version of a family favourite.

🕐 1 hour 5 mins   ◔ Cuts into 12

- 75ml/2½fl oz rapeseed oil, plus extra for the tin
- 175g/6oz self-raising flour
- 1½ tsp baking powder
- 50g/2oz ground almonds
- 50g/2oz polenta (cornmeal)
- finely grated zest 2 lemons
- 140g/5oz golden caster sugar
- 2 large eggs
- 225g/8oz natural yogurt

FOR THE LEMON SYRUP
- 85g/3oz caster sugar
- juice 2 lemons (about 5 tbsp)

1 Heat oven to 180C/160C fan/gas 4. Lightly oil a 20cm round deep cake tin and line the base with baking parchment. For the cake, put the flour, baking powder, ground almonds and polenta in a large mixing bowl. Stir in the lemon zest and sugar, then make a dip in the centre. Beat the eggs in a bowl, then stir in the yogurt. Tip this mixture along with the oil into the dip then briefly and gently stir with a large metal spoon so everything is just combined, without overmixing.

2 Spoon the mixture into the tin and level the top. Bake for 40 mins or until a skewer inserted into the centre of the cake comes out clean. Cover loosely with foil for the final 5–10 mins if it starts to brown too quickly.

3 While the cake cooks, make the lemon syrup. Tip the caster sugar into a small saucepan with the lemon juice and 75ml water. Heat over a medium heat, stirring occasionally, until the sugar has dissolved. Raise the heat, boil for 4 mins until slightly reduced and syrupy, then remove from the heat.

4 Remove the cake from the oven and let it cool briefly in the tin. While it is still warm, turn it out of the tin, peel off the lining paper and sit the cake on a wire rack set over a baking tray or similar. Use a skewer to make lots of small holes all over the top of the cake. Slowly spoon over half the lemon syrup and let it soak in. Spoon over the rest in the same way, brushing the edges and sides of the cake too with the last of the syrup.

PER SLICE 243 kcals, fat 10g, saturates 1.5g, carbs 35g, sugars 21g, fibre 0.9g, protein 5g, salt 0.34g

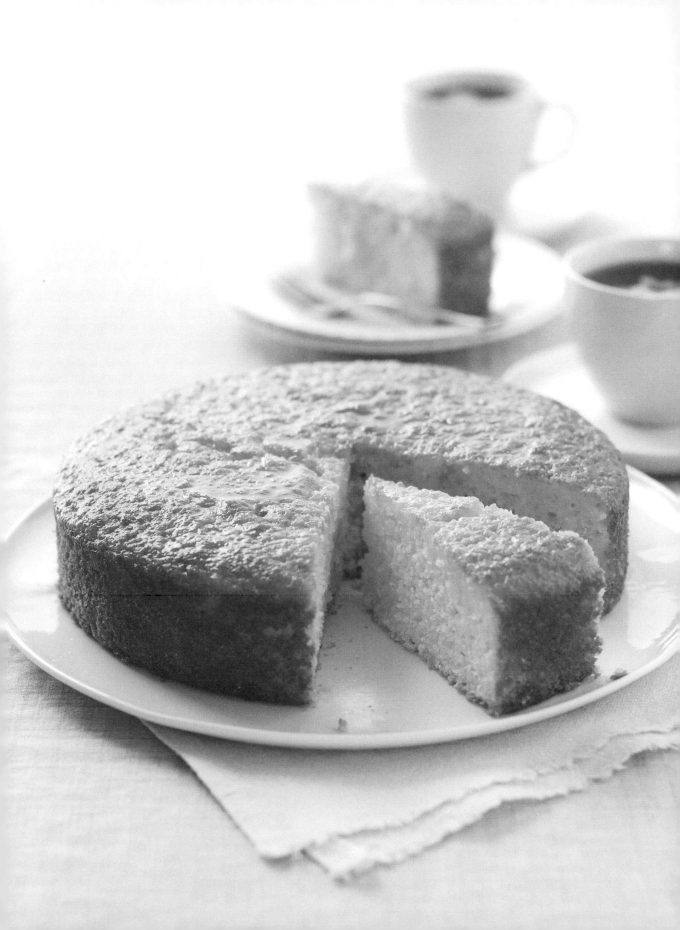

Lighter Victoria Sandwich

The classic teatime sponge cake is given a healthy makeover to halve the fat and reduce the sugar, without losing any of the taste.

🕐 45 mins   ◔ Cuts into 8 slices

- 2 tbsp rapeseed oil, plus extra for the tin
- 175g/6oz self-raising flour
- 1½ tsp baking powder
- 140g/5oz golden caster sugar
- 25g/1oz ground almonds
- 2 large eggs
- 175g/6oz natural yogurt
- 2–3 drops vanilla extract
- 25g/1oz butter, melted
- 4 tbsp raspberry conserve
- ½ tsp icing sugar, to decorate

1 Heat oven to 180C/160C fan/gas 4. Lightly oil 2 x 18cm sandwich cake tins (preferably loose-bottomed) and line the bases with baking parchment. Tip the flour, baking powder, caster sugar and ground almonds into a large mixing bowl, then make a well in the centre. Beat the eggs in a bowl, then stir in the yogurt and vanilla. Pour this mixture, along with the melted butter and oil, into the dry mixture and stir briefly together with a large metal spoon until well combined.

2 Divide the mixture evenly between the 2 tins and level the tops. Bake both cakes, side by side, for 20 mins until risen and beginning to come away slightly from the edges of the tins.

3 Remove the cakes from the oven and loosen the sides with a round-bladed knife. Let the cakes cool briefly in the tins, then turn them out. If the tins are loose-bottomed, an easy way is to sit the tin on an upturned jam jar and let the outer ring of the tin drop down. Peel off the lining paper and sit the cakes on a wire rack. Leave until completely cold.

4 Put one of the cakes on a serving plate and spread over the conserve. Put the other cake on top and sift over the icing sugar, or make a pattern with a paper cut out and then dusting.

PER SLICE 263 kcals, fat 9g, saturates 3g, carbs 39g, sugars 24g, fibre 2g, protein 6g, salt 0.6g

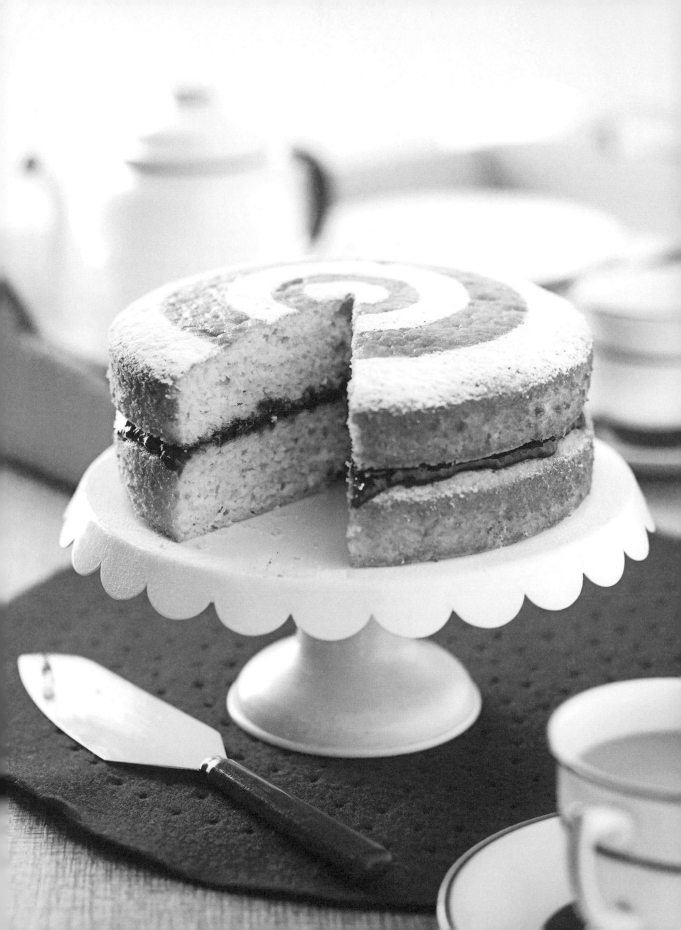

Lighter Gingerbread

This dark and sticky cake is made healthier with naturally sweet dates, buttermilk and plenty of cinnamon and fresh and dried ginger.

🕐 1 hour 15 mins   ◔ Cuts into 21 pieces

- 140g/5oz dried pitted whole dates, chopped into small pieces
- 75ml/2½fl oz rapeseed oil, plus a few drops for greasing
- 75g/2½oz black treacle
- 50g/2oz maple syrup
- 1 tsp finely grated fresh ginger
- 1 large egg
- 175ml/6fl oz buttermilk or a mix of milk and yogurt
- 250g/9oz plain flour
- 1 tsp bicarbonate of soda
- 1 tbsp ground ginger
- ½ tsp ground cinnamon
- 50g/2oz dark muscovado sugar

1 Put the dates in a small bowl and pour over 125ml of boiling water. Leave to cool for 30 mins. Lightly oil a 28 x 19 x 3cm traybake tin, then line the base with baking parchment.

2 Meanwhile, put the oil, black treacle, maple syrup and freshly grated ginger in a bowl and beat together with a fork to mix well. Set aside. Beat the egg in a small bowl and stir in the buttermilk. In a large bowl, mix the flour with the bicarbonate of soda, ground ginger, cinnamon and sugar – rub the mixture between your fingers to break down any lumpy bits of sugar. Heat oven to 160C/140C fan/gas 3.

3 Blend the dates and their liquid to a thick purée in a small food processor. Pour the egg, the dates and the treacle mixture into the bowl with the flour. Stir together briefly with a wooden spoon just until well mixed – the mixture will be soft like a thick batter. Pour it into the lined tin, gently level the mixture and bake for 40–45 mins. To test if it's done, insert a skewer in the centre – if the skewer comes out clean with no uncooked mixture on it, and the cake feels firm but springy to the touch, it should be done.

4 Leave in the tin for a few mins before removing to a wire rack, peeling off the parchment and leaving to cool completely. If you can wait, wrap it well in parchment, then foil. Leave for a day before cutting, as it will become stickier – it will keep moist for 3–4 days.

PER PIECE 116 kcals, fat 4g, saturates 0.4g, carbs 18g, sugars 8g, fibre 0.7g, protein 2g, salt 0.2g

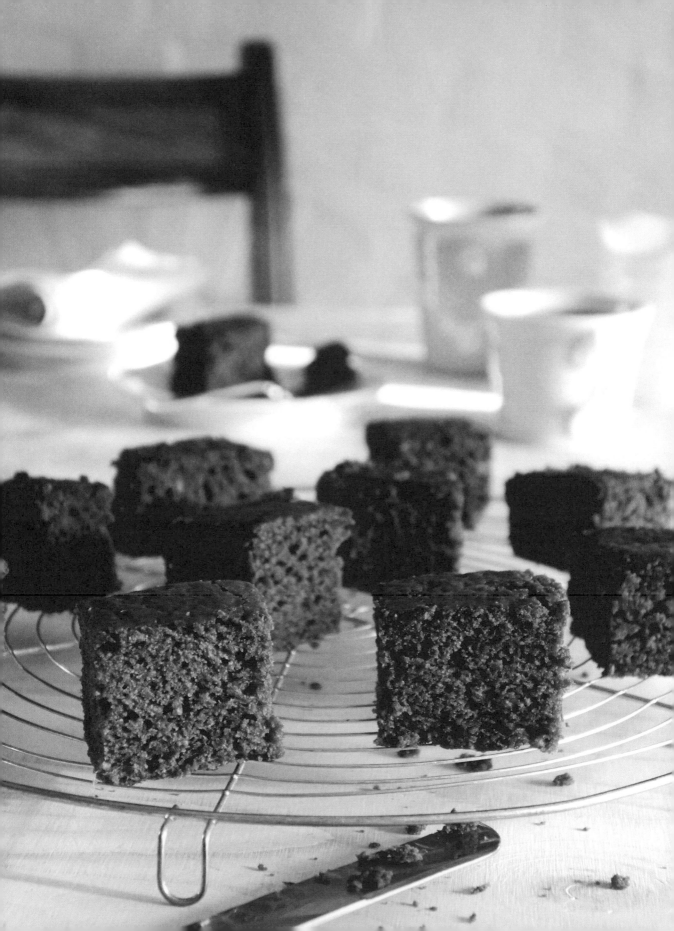

Lighter Spiced Carrot Cake

This moist classic traybake uses sweet potato for natural sweetness to reduce the sugar and a lower-fat frosting.

🕐 1 hour   ◔ Cuts into 15 squares

- 125ml/4fl oz rapeseed oil, plus a little extra for greasing
- 300g/11oz wholemeal flour
- 2 tsp baking powder
- 1 tsp bicarbonate of soda
- 1 tbsp mixed spice
- 100g/4oz dark soft brown sugar
- 140g/5oz carrots, grated
- 140g/5oz sweet potatoes, peeled and grated
- 200g/7oz sultanas
- 2 large eggs
- 4 tbsp maple syrup
- juice 2 oranges

FOR THE ICING
- 200g/7oz quark
- 50g/2oz fromage frais
- 3 tbsp icing sugar, sifted
- zest 1 orange

1 Heat oven to 180C/160C fan/gas 4. Grease and line a 20 x 30cm traybake tin with baking parchment. Mix together the flour, baking powder, bicarb, spice and sugar in a big mixing bowl. Stir in the grated carrots, sweet potatoes and sultanas. In a jug, whisk together the eggs, rapeseed oil, syrup and juice from 1 orange. Tip the wet ingredients into the bowl and stir to combine, then scrape into the tin. Bake for 25–30 mins until a skewer poked in comes out clean. Prick all over with a skewer and drizzle over the remaining orange juice. Cool in the tin.

2 Once cool, make the icing. Stir the quark with a spoon to make it a bit smoother, then fold in the fromage frais, icing sugar and orange zest. Spread all over the cake and slice into squares to eat.

PER SQUARE 269 kcals, fat 10g, saturates 1g, carbs 38g, sugars 25g, fibre 3g, protein 6g, salt 0.4g

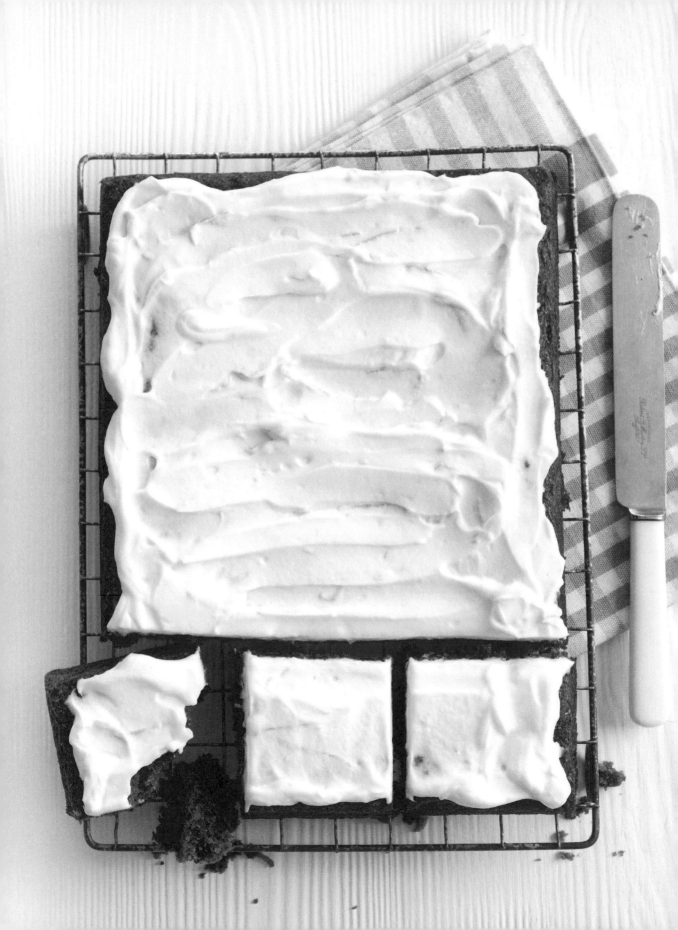

Lighter Bakewell Tart

This version has less fat and sugar than the original and uses fresh raspberries to cut back on the amount of jam used.

🕐 1 hour 15 mins   🥧 Cuts into 8 slices

- 200g/7oz shop-bought shortcrust pastry
- plain flour, for dusting
- 100g/4oz fresh raspberries
- 1 tbsp raspberry conserve or jam
- 1 tbsp flaked almonds
- 1 heaped tbsp icing sugar

FOR THE FILLING

- 50g/2oz ground almonds
- 50g/2oz polenta (cornmeal)
- 50g/2oz golden caster sugar, plus 2 tsp
- ½ tsp baking powder
- 2 medium eggs
- 100g/4oz natural yogurt
- scant ½ tsp almond extract (optional)
- 2 tbsp rapeseed oil

1 Heat oven to 200C/180C fan/gas 6. Thinly roll out the pastry on a lightly floured surface. Line a 20cm round x 4cm deep fluted flan tin with the pastry, easing it into the tin and the flutes carefully so you don't stretch it. Roll a rolling pin over the top of the tin to trim off any excess pastry. Prick the base lightly with a fork. Put the tin on a baking sheet.

2 Line the pastry with foil and baking beans and bake for 12 mins until the pastry is set. Meanwhile, to make the filling, heat a small, dry non-stick pan, tip in the ground almonds and gently heat, stirring often, for 2–3 mins to lightly brown. Transfer to a medium-sized mixing bowl to cool. Remove the foil and beans from the pastry case and bake for 5 mins more until pale golden. Remove and reduce oven to 180C/160C fan/gas 4.

3 Using a fork, roughly mash the raspberries in a small bowl with the jam, so they are still in small pieces and not completely mashed. Evenly spread the raspberry mixture over the pastry base. Put the polenta, sugar and baking powder in the mixing bowl with the almonds and stir to combine. Make a well in the centre. Beat the eggs in a bowl, then beat in the yogurt and almond extract, if using. Tip this mixture, along with the oil, into the dry ingredients, and briefly and gently stir together with a large metal spoon so everything is just combined – don't overmix.

4 Pour the almond filling over the raspberry mixture and scatter the flaked almonds over the top. Bake for 30 mins or until the top is risen and pale golden. Cool slightly, then remove from the tin.

5 Mix the icing sugar with a few drops of cold water to make a thick-ish icing, then use a teaspoon to drizzle it over the cooled tart. The tart is even softer when eaten the next day. Will keep in an airtight container for up to 3 days.

PER SLICE 280 kcals, fat 16g, saturates 4g, carbs 27g, sugars 13g, fibre 1g, protein 6g, salt 0.4g

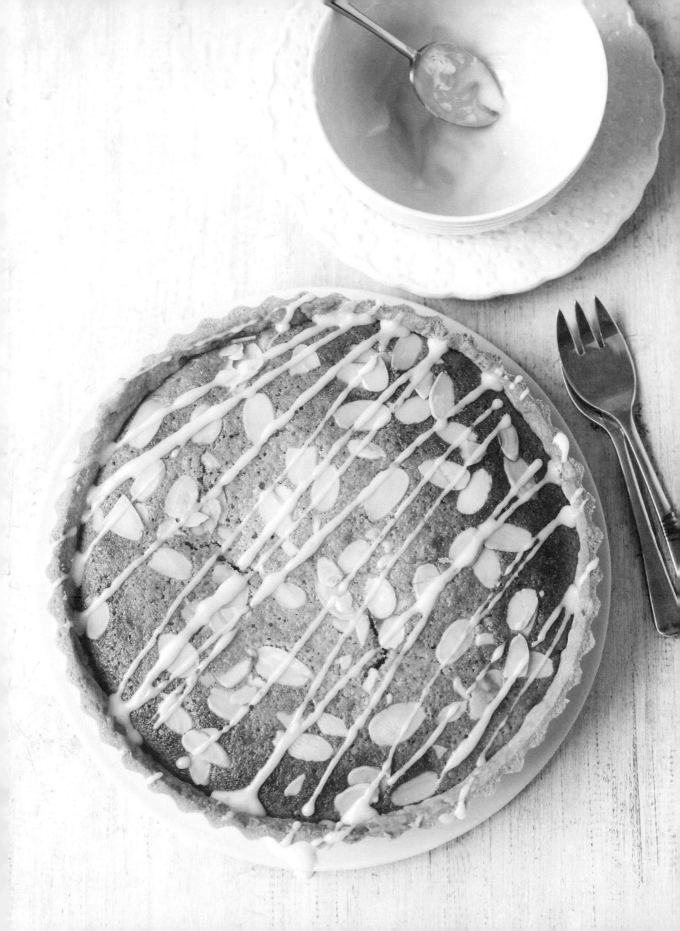

Eggless Chocolate Beetroot Blitz & Bake Cake

Healthier than your average chocolate cake, this rich dark bake is lighter on the calorie count, too.

⏱ 1 hour 20 mins   🥧 10-12

- 100ml/3½fl oz rapeseed oil, plus extra for greasing
- 175g/6oz (drained weight) vacuum-packed beetroot (not in vinegar)
- 175g/6oz dark soft brown sugar
- 200g/7oz self-raising flour
- 1 tbsp baking powder
- 50g/2oz cocoa powder
- 200g/7oz 0%-fat natural yogurt
- 2 tsp vanilla extract

FOR THE ICING
- 100g/4oz icing sugar
- 50g/2oz dark chocolate (at least 80% cocoa solids)
- 1 tbsp cocoa
- 3 tbsp skimmed milk
- dark chocolate shavings, to serve (optional)

1 Heat oven to 180C/160C fan/gas 4 and boil the kettle. Grease and line a deep 20cm springform cake tin with baking parchment. Tip the beetroot into a food processor and whizz to a purée. Add the remaining ingredients, along with ¼ tsp salt, and blend until well combined. Scrape into the cake tin, level the surface and bake for 50 mins–1 hr or until a skewer comes out clean.

2 Leave the cake to cool in the tin while you make the icing. Put the ingredients in a small saucepan, heat and whisk until smooth. Cool for 20 mins.

3 Flip the cake onto a wire rack, flat-side up. Pour over the icing and leave to cool completely. Sprinkle with dark chocolate shavings (if using), then serve.

PER SLICE (12) 276 kcals, fat 11g, saturates 2g, carbs 39g, sugars 26g, fibre 2g, protein 5g, salt 0.5g

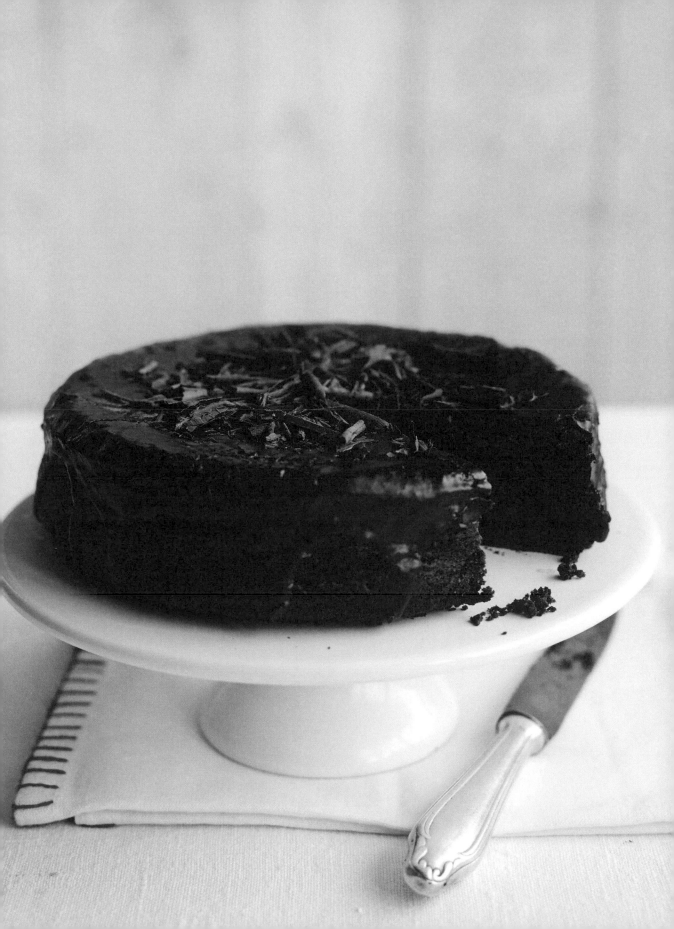

Makeover Blueberry Muffins

A deliciously light version of a classic muffin that contains virtually no saturated fat. You need an extra-ripe banana for this – so it's a good way to use them up from the fruit bowl.

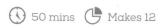 50 mins Makes 12

- 5 tbsp rapeseed oil
- 225g/8oz self-raising flour
- 115g/4oz wholemeal flour
- 2 tsp baking powder
- zest ½ lemon and 1 tsp juice
- 85g/3oz golden caster sugar
- 50g/2oz light muscovado sugar
- 1 small very ripe banana with black skin (about 85g/3oz peeled weight)
- 1 egg
- 284ml pot buttermilk
- 225g/8oz fresh blueberries

1 Heat oven to 200C/180C fan/gas 6. Use 1 tsp oil to lightly oil a 12-hole muffin tin (or use paper cases). Mix both flours with the baking powder and lemon zest. Reserve 1 tbsp caster sugar, then stir the rest into the flour with the muscovado.

2 Mash the banana well. In another bowl beat the egg, then stir in the banana, buttermilk and oil. Using a large metal spoon, very lightly stir into the flour mix, just to combine. Over-mixing will make the muffins tough. Toss in the blueberries and give just a few turns of the spoon to carefully stir them in without crushing.

3 Spoon the mixture into the tin – each hole should be very full. Bake for 20–25 mins until risen and golden.

4 Mix the reserved caster sugar with the lemon juice. When the muffins are done, remove from the oven, then brush with the sugar and lemon mixture while they are still hot. Gently loosen the edges of each muffin with a knife, then leave in the tin for 15 mins to cool a little as they're very delicate while hot. Remove to a wire rack. Best eaten the day of making, but will keep for up to 2 days.

PER MUFFIN 206 kcals, fat 6g, saturates 1g, carbs 36g, sugars 16g, fibre 2g, protein 5g, salt 0.43g

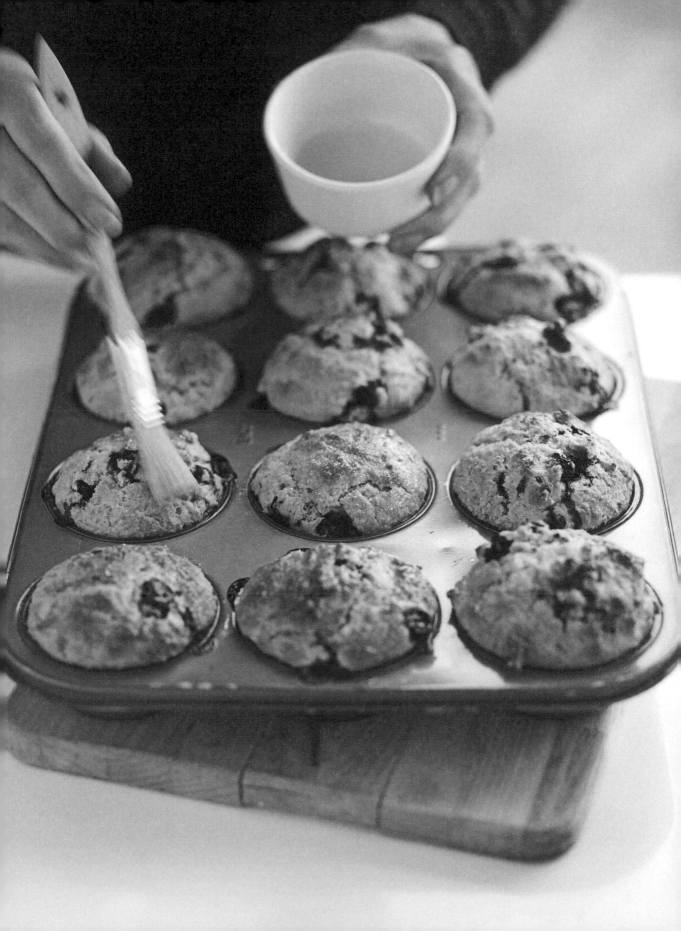

Lighter Apple & Pear Pie

A crispy filo top with a deep layer of spiced apple and pears makes this a great family dessert for the weekend.

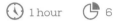 1 hour 6

- 6 eating apples (we used Braeburn)
- 4 ripe pears
- juice and zest 1 lemon
- 3 tbsp maple syrup
- 1 tsp mixed spice
- 1 tbsp cornflour
- 4 filo sheets
- 4 tsp rapeseed oil
- 25g/1oz flaked almonds

TO SERVE
- custard (made with custard powder and skimmed milk), fat-free Greek yogurt or low-fat frozen vanilla yogurt

1 Peel, core and chop the apples and pears into large pieces and throw into a big saucepan with the lemon juice, syrup, mixed spice and 200ml water. Bring to a simmer with the lid on, then take off the lid and cook, stirring, for about 5 mins until the apple is softening. Use a slotted spoon to scoop out three-quarters of the fruit chunks and put into a pie dish.

2 Cover and cook the remaining fruit for another 4–5 mins until soft, then mash with a potato masher. Mix 1 tbsp of this with the cornflour to a smooth paste, then add back to the pan and bring back to a simmer, stirring, to thicken the sauce. Pour over the fruit in the pie dish and stir together. Heat oven to 180C/160C fan/gas 4.

3 Lay out your sheets of filo and brush all over with oil – 1 tsp should be enough for 1 sheet. Scatter over the almonds and press to stick to the pastry, then crumple up each sheet as you lift it on top of the fruit. Bake for 20–25 mins until the pastry is browned and crisp. Serve straight away with custard, yogurt or frozen yogurt.

PER SERVING 225 kcals, fat 5g, saturates none, carbs 43g, sugars 25g, fibre 5g, protein 4g, salt 0.3g

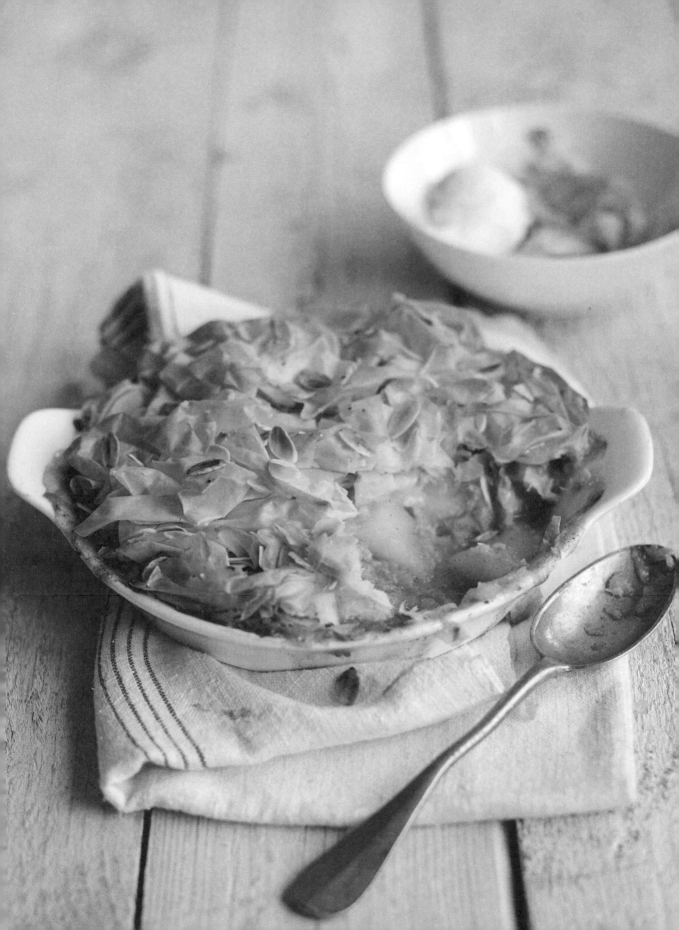

Lighter Creamy Vanilla Rice Pudding

Rich and comforting, but without the cream this is low-fat and full of calcium.

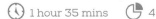 1 hour 35 mins 4

- ¼ tsp butter, for greasing
- 85g/3oz short-grain (pudding) rice
- 1 tbsp light muscovado sugar
- 2 tsp golden caster sugar
- 700ml/1¼ pints semi-skimmed milk, plus 50ml/2fl oz
- ½ vanilla pod or ½ tsp vanilla extract
- 3 tbsp half-fat crème fraîche
- fresh raspberries, to serve (optional)

1 Heat oven to 150C/130C fan/gas 2. Grease a 1.2-litre (about 5cm deep) ovenproof baking dish and stand it on a baking tray. Tip the rice into a pan with both the sugars and all the milk. Split the ½ vanilla pod horizontally, scrape out the seeds into the pan and drop in the pod or add the extract. Heat the milk, whisking. As it is about to come to the boil, immediately remove from the heat. Pour the mixture into the dish, scraping out all the rice and seeds from the bottom of the pan.

2 Bake for 30 mins, then remove and stir. Return the pudding to the oven for another 30 mins. Stir again and return for a further 25–30 mins until the rice is cooked and has absorbed enough of the milk to give the mixture a creamy consistency.

3 Remove the pudding, let it sit for 1–2 mins, then stir in the crème fraîche to make it extra creamy. Serve with fresh raspberries, if you like.

PER SERVING 204 kcals, fat 6g, saturates 4g, carbs 29g, sugars 12g, fibre 0.6g, protein 8g, salt 0.2g

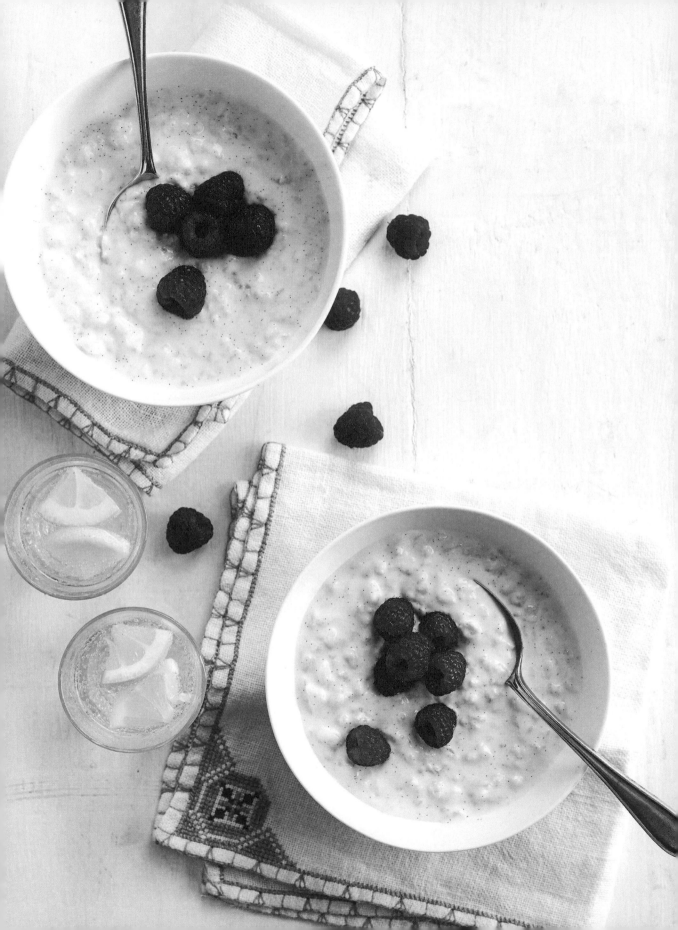

Honey Nut Crunch Pears

A quick throw-together dessert from the storecupboard.

15 mins 4

- 4 ripe pears
- knob of butter
- ½ tsp mixed spice
- 2 tbsp clear honey
- 50g/2oz cornflakes
- 25g/1oz toasted flaked almonds
- ice cream, to serve

1 Heat oven to 200C/180C fan/gas 6. Cut the pears in half lengthways, take out the core then top with a small knob of butter and a sprinkling of the mixed spice. Sit the pears in a shallow baking dish, then roast for 5 mins until starting to soften. Meanwhile, heat the honey and another knob of butter in a large bowl in the microwave for 30 secs. Toss with the cornflakes and nuts.

2 Take the pears out of the oven, then top with the cornflake mix. Cook for another 5 mins or until the cornflakes take on a rich golden colour. Allow to cool for a few mins (the cornflakes crisp up again as they cool), then serve warm with ice cream.

PER SERVING 179 kcals, fat 6g, saturates 1g, carbs 31g, sugars 21g, fibre 4g, protein 3g, salt 0.37g

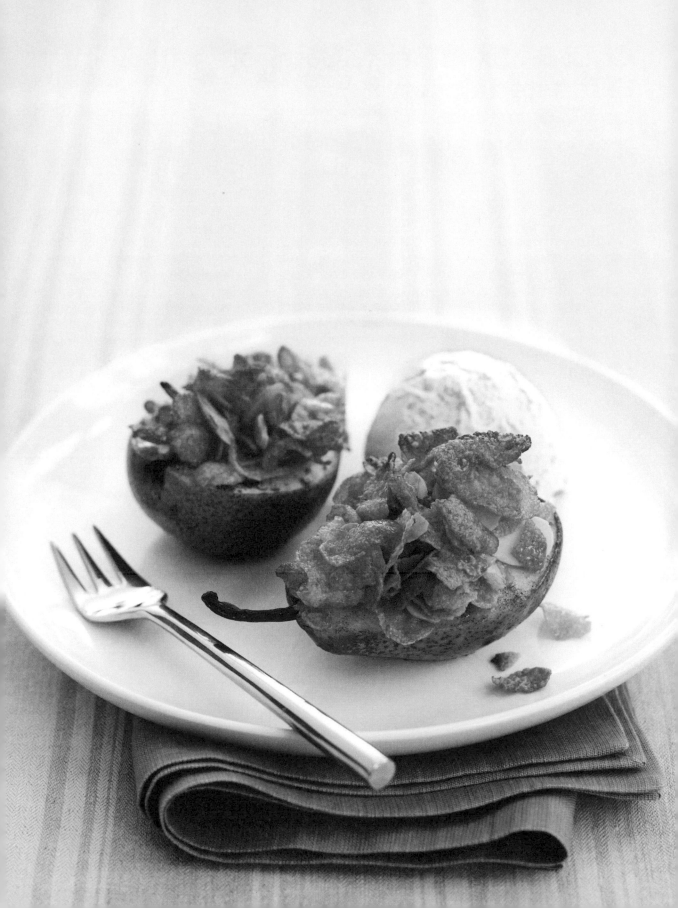

Chia & Mixed Berry Compote with Yogurt & Toasted Coconut

High-protein, mineral-rich chia seeds are used in these healthy desserts that can also be served for breakfast. Any leftover seeds can be added to porridge or homemade breads.

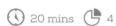 20 mins · 4

- 25g/1oz unsweetened coconut shavings
- 275g pack frozen mixed red berries, such as forest fruits or summer berries
- 6 tbsp orange or mixed fruit juice, or water
- honey, to sweeten
- 2 tbsp chia seeds
- 300g/11oz low-fat Greek yogurt

1 Heat oven to 200C/180C fan/gas 6. Scatter the coconut over a baking sheet and bake in the oven for 3–4 mins or until the edges are just turning toasty brown. Leave to cool.

2 Put the frozen fruits in a pan with the fruit juice or water and very gently heat until the fruits have collapsed. Sweeten to taste, stir in the chia seeds and leave to cool – the juices will thicken as the chia seeds swell.

3 In 4 small tumblers or pots, top a layer of fruit with yogurt or add several alternating layers, starting with fruit and ending with yogurt. Sprinkle with the coconut and serve.

PER SERVING 152 kcals, fat 7g, saturates 4g, carbs 15g, sugars 11g, fibre 4g, protein 6g, salt 0.2g

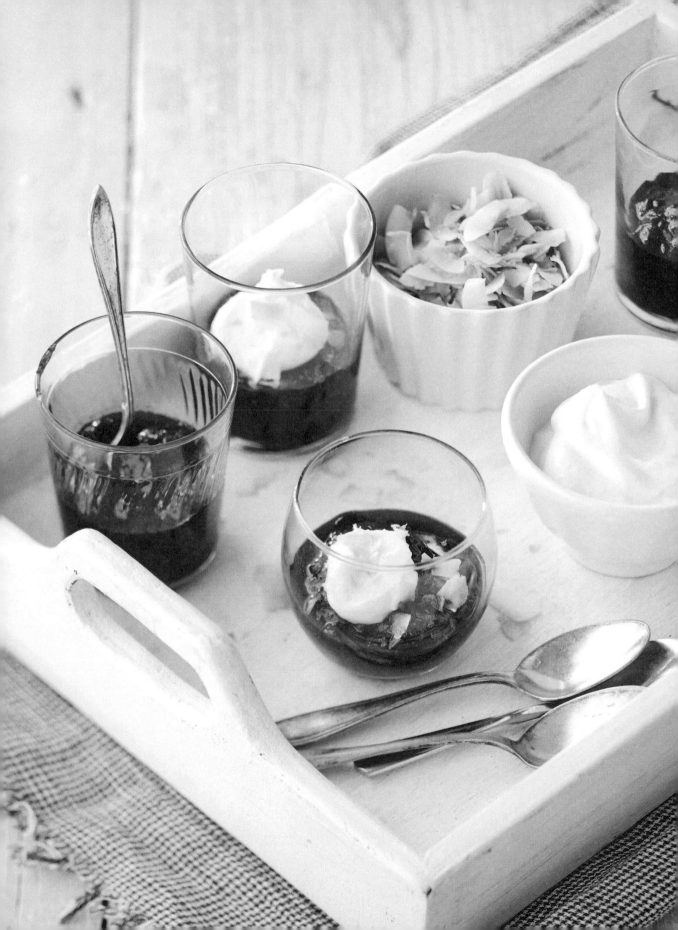

Lighter Crème Brûlée

The secret to this healthier version is to make sure that the custard is nice and thick, as unlike a normal crème brûlée recipe, the custard isn't baked afterwards.

🕐 40 mins, plus overnight chilling 🥧 4

- 4 tbsp golden caster sugar
- 1 tbsp custard powder
- 1 tbsp cornflour
- 200ml/7fl oz semi-skimmed milk
- 2 large egg yolks
- 125ml/4fl oz single cream
- 1 vanilla pod or 1 tsp vanilla extract
- 140g/5oz half-fat crème fraîche

1 Stir 2 tbsp of the sugar, the custard powder and cornflour in a medium bowl with 2 tbsp of the milk to a smooth paste. Beat in the egg yolks with a fork until well combined. Pour the remaining milk into a pan, then pour in the cream. Slit the vanilla pod lengthways and scrape the seeds into the milk. Drop the pod into the pan and bring just to the boil – as soon as a few bubbles rise to the surface, remove from the heat.

2 Slowly pour and stir the hot milk into the cornflour mix, including the vanilla pod, making sure the yolks are well blended in. Transfer to a clean pan. Cook over a low heat, stirring continuously with a wooden spoon, for about 15–20 mins until the mixture is very thick – when you drag the spoon across the bottom of the pan it should leave a clean line. It should be much thicker after about 10 mins, but keep stirring until the mixture has thickened and looks like softly whipped cream. Keep adjusting the heat so that the mixture does not come to the boil or overheat, as it may curdle and become lumpy. If this happens, beat the mixture smooth with a wire whisk.

3 Remove from the heat, transfer to a bowl and cool for 15–20 mins, stirring occasionally to prevent a skin forming. Remove the vanilla pod, if using. Stir in the crème fraîche and divide the mixture between 4 small ramekins (125–150ml capacity each). Level the mixtures, then chill, uncovered, overnight. Not covering them means a thin skin forms on top which supports the caramel.

4 Before serving, spoon the remaining sugar over the top of each custard (allow 1½ tsp per ramekin) and smooth with the back of the spoon. To caramelise, hold the blowtorch just above the sugar and keep it moving until evenly caramelised (do it quickly or you will heat the custard too much). If the custard has softened slightly, put the ramekins in the fridge for 5–10 mins to firm up. Serve while the caramel is still brittle.

PER SERVING 257 kcals, fat 15g, saturates 9g, carbs 25g, sugars 19g, fibre none, protein 5g, salt 0.2g

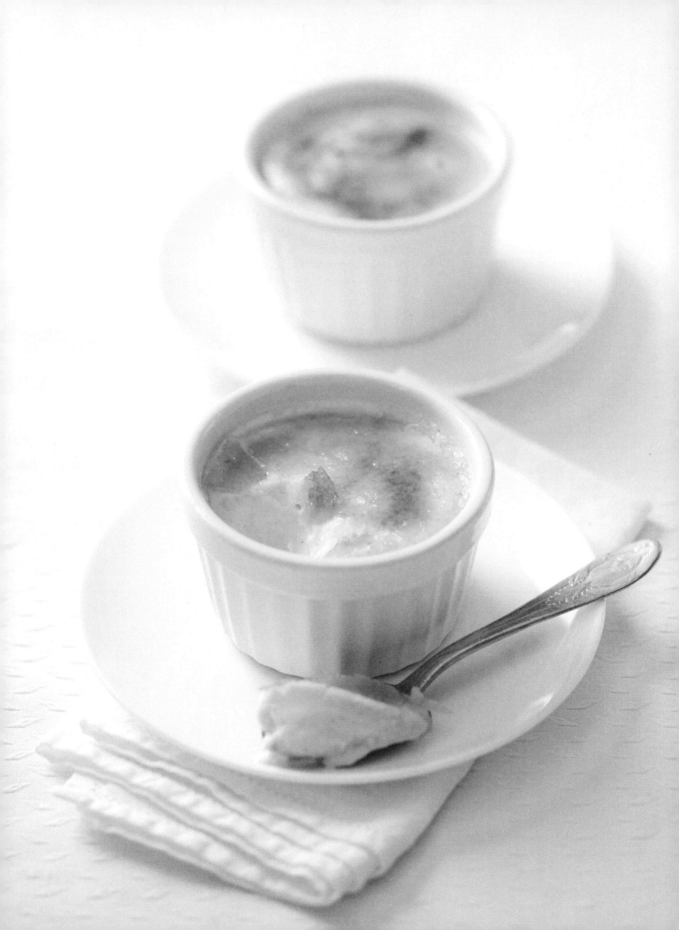

Peach Crumble

This low-calorie dessert made using tinned peaches will give you 2 of your 5 a day.

🕐 45 mins 🥧 6

- 3 x 410g cans peach slices in juice
- zest 1 lemon, plus juice ½
- 2 tbsp maple syrup
- 140g/5oz plain flour
- 50g/2oz porridge oats
- 25g/1oz cold butter, grated

1 Heat oven to 200C/180C fan/gas 6. Drain the peaches, but reserve the juice. Tip the peaches into a deep baking dish, roughly 20 x 30cm. Scatter over the lemon zest and juice and 1 tbsp of the syrup, then toss everything together.

2 In a bowl, combine the flour, oats, butter, remaining syrup and 4 tbsp of the reserved peach juice. Mix together, first with a spoon, then with your fingers, until you have a rough crumbly mixture. Scatter over the peaches, then bake for 35 mins until golden and crunchy on top.

PER SERVING 202 kcals, fat 4g, saturates 2g, carbs 36g, sugars 14g, fibre 3g, protein 4g, salt 0.1g

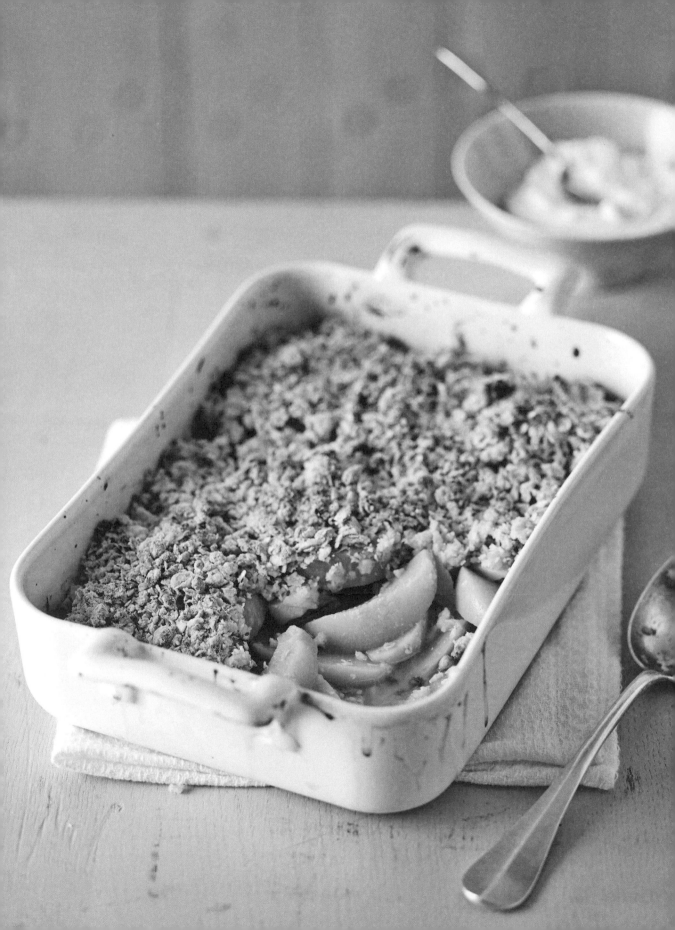

Chocolate Sponge with Hot Chocolate Custard

Easy to make and low-fat, this is a pudding for a crowd when you want to entertain. The sugar content is still quite high, though, so eat in moderation.

🕐 1 hour 20 mins 🥧 12-15

- 300g/11oz stoned dates, chopped
- 6 large eggs, separated
- 225g/8oz light muscovado sugar
- 200g/7oz wholemeal flour
- 2 tsp baking powder
- 100g/4oz cocoa

FOR THE CUSTARD
- 5 tbsp custard powder
- 5 tbsp light muscovado sugar
- 50g/2oz cocoa
- 1.2 litres/2 pints skimmed milk

1 Cover the dates with boiling water and set aside to soften for 30 mins.
2 Heat oven to 160C/140C fan/gas 3 and line a 20 x 30cm baking tin with baking parchment. Drain the dates, reserving the liquid, then whizz them to a purée with 200ml of the soaking liquid.
3 Beat the egg whites in a large bowl with an electric whisk until stiff peaks hold on the end of your whisk. Add half the sugar and beat until thick and glossy.
4 In another bowl, beat the yolks and remaining sugar until pale. Whisk in the mashed date mixture, then fold into the egg white mixture until well combined. Mix the flour, baking powder and cocoa. Sprinkle over the wet mixture and very gently fold in until well combined. Gently scrape into the tin and spread to the edges. Bake for 35–40 mins until a skewer poked in comes out clean.
5 Meanwhile, mix the custard powder, sugar and cocoa together in a saucepan. Stir in dribbles of milk until you get a smooth paste. Gradually add more milk until it's all incorporated with no lumps. Put over a medium heat and warm, stirring constantly, until thick and just bubbling.
6 Cut the warm cake into squares and pour over the hot chocolate custard to serve.

PER SERVING (15) 298kcals, fat 4g, saturates 2g, carbs 52g, sugars 38g, fibre 4g, protein 10g, salt 0.4g

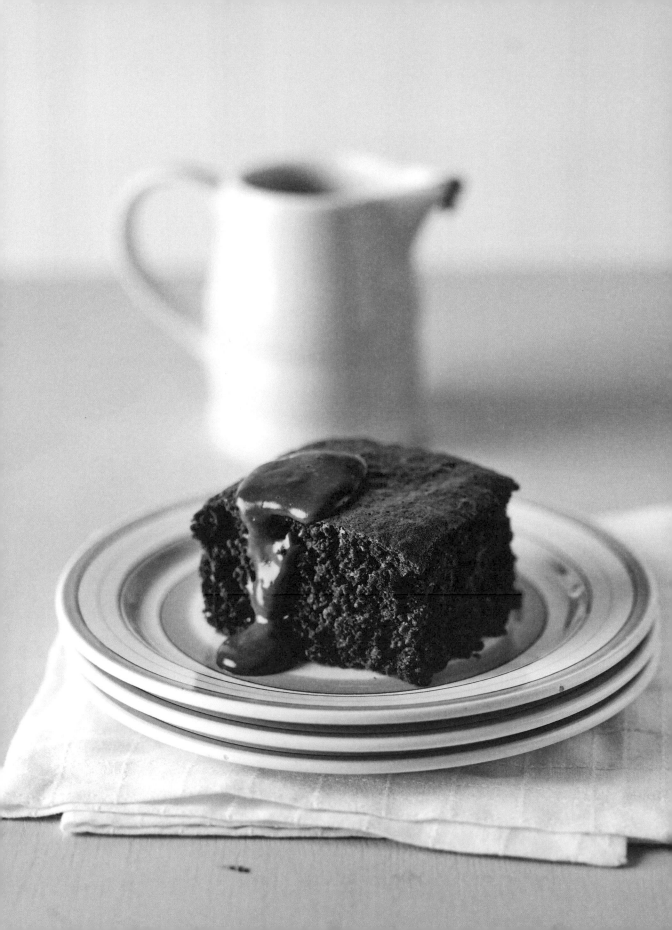

Oeufs au Lait

These little French vanilla custard puddings are deliciously creamy and surprisingly low in fat. They will keep in the fridge for up to 2 days.

🕐 40 minutes, plus chilling ◔ 4

- butter, for greasing
- 425ml/¾ pint milk
- 85g/3oz caster sugar
- 1 tsp vanilla extract
- 2 eggs

1 Butter four ramekins, about 150ml/¼ pint each. Heat oven to 160C/140C fan/gas 3. Have a roasting tin ready and put the kettle on.
2 Pour the milk into a pan with the sugar and vanilla. Bring gently to the boil, stirring to dissolve the sugar. Remove from the heat and cool for a few mins.
3 In a large bowl, beat the eggs until frothy. Slowly whisk in the milk. Set the ramekins in the roasting tin and divide the custard among them. Pour hot water around the ramekins to come halfway up the sides. Bake for 20 mins until just set, then cool and chill before serving.

PER SERVING 181 kcals, fat 5g, saturates 2g, carbs 28g, sugars 23g, fibre none, protein 7g, salt 0.23g

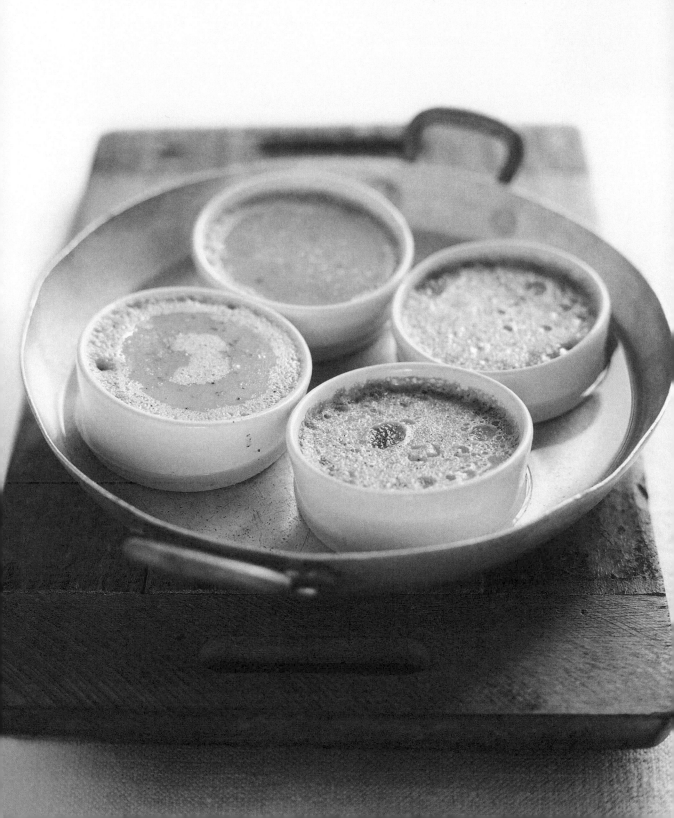

Cherry & Raspberry Gratin

Make the most of the summer fruits when they're in season. The contrast of sweet vanilla with the tart cherries and raspberries works very well in this healthy pud.

 25 minutes, plus infusing 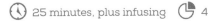 4

- 200ml/7fl oz milk
- 1 vanilla pod, split lengthways or 1 tsp vanilla extract
- 2 eggs, separated
- 4 tbsp caster sugar
- 1 tbsp plain flour
- squeeze of lemon juice
- 300g/10oz stoned cherries
- 300g/10oz raspberries

1 Heat the milk and vanilla pod in a pan until nearly boiling, then leave to infuse for 10–15 mins – if using extract you can use the milk straight away. Whisk together the egg yolks with 2 tbsp of the sugar until pale and light, then whisk in the flour to make a paste. Whisk in the warm milk. Pour the mixture into a pan, then cook for 3–5 mins until thick. Pour through a sieve into a large bowl, discarding the vanilla pod, if using. Leave to cool.

2 Whisk the egg whites until stiff peaks form then add the remaining sugar, a little at a time, whisking well between each addition, until the mixture is thick and glossy. Stir the lemon juice into the custard mix. Add a third of the meringue to the custard and stir. Repeat with the remaining meringue.

3 Scatter the fruit into a large, shallow heatproof dish. Put under a medium grill for 3–5 mins to soften. Spoon over the custard mix then grill for 3 mins until the topping is golden.

PER SERVING 218 kcals, fat 6g, saturates 2g, carbs 33g, sugars 30g, fibre 3g, protein 9g, salt 0.22g

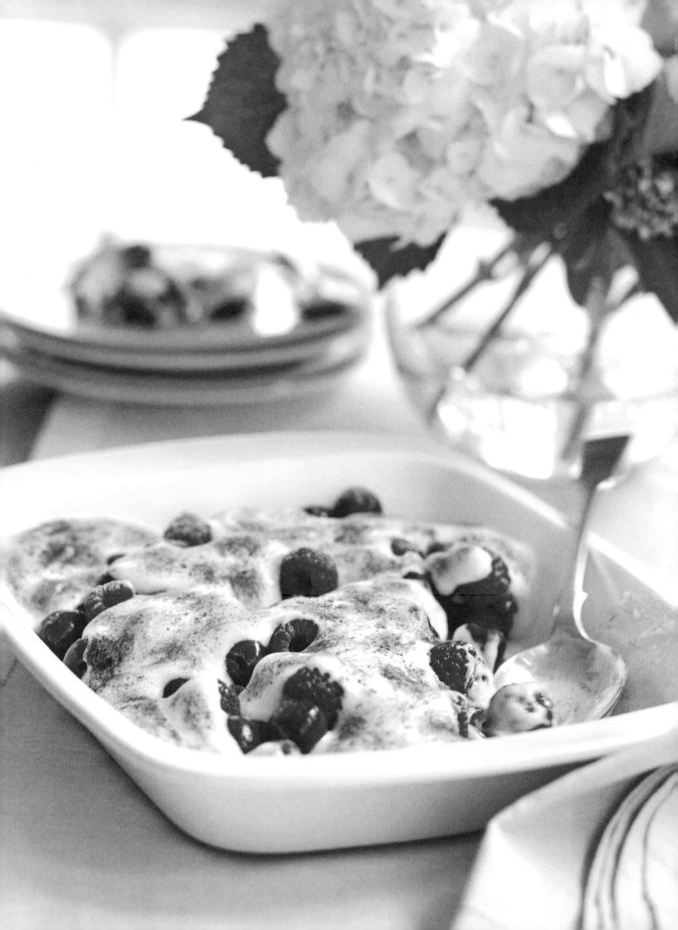

Apricot & Raspberry Tart

Filo pastry is a low-fat alternative to richer pastries like puff and shortcrust, however it needs to be brushed with a little butter as it is layered up.

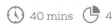 40 mins 4

- 3 large sheets filo pastry (or 6 small)
- 2 tbsp butter, melted
- 3 tbsp apricot conserve
- 6 ripe apricots, stoned and roughly sliced
- 85g/3oz raspberries
- 2 tsp caster sugar

1 Let the filo come to room temperature for about 10 mins before use. Put a baking tray into the oven and heat oven to 200C/180C fan/gas 6.

2 Brush each large sheet of filo with melted butter, layer on top of each other, then fold in half so you have a smaller rectangle 6 layers thick. If using small sheets just stack them on top of each other. Fold in the edges of the pastry base to make a 2cm border, then spread the apricot conserve inside the border. Carefully slide the pastry base onto the hot baking tray and bake for 5 mins.

3 Remove from the oven, arrange the apricots over the tart and brush with any leftover melted butter. Bake for another 10 mins, then scatter on the raspberries and sprinkle with sugar. Bake for a final 10 mins until the pastry is golden brown and crisp.

PER SERVING 150 kcals, fat 7g, saturates 4g, carbs 22g, sugars 18g, fibre 2g, protein 2g, salt 0.33g

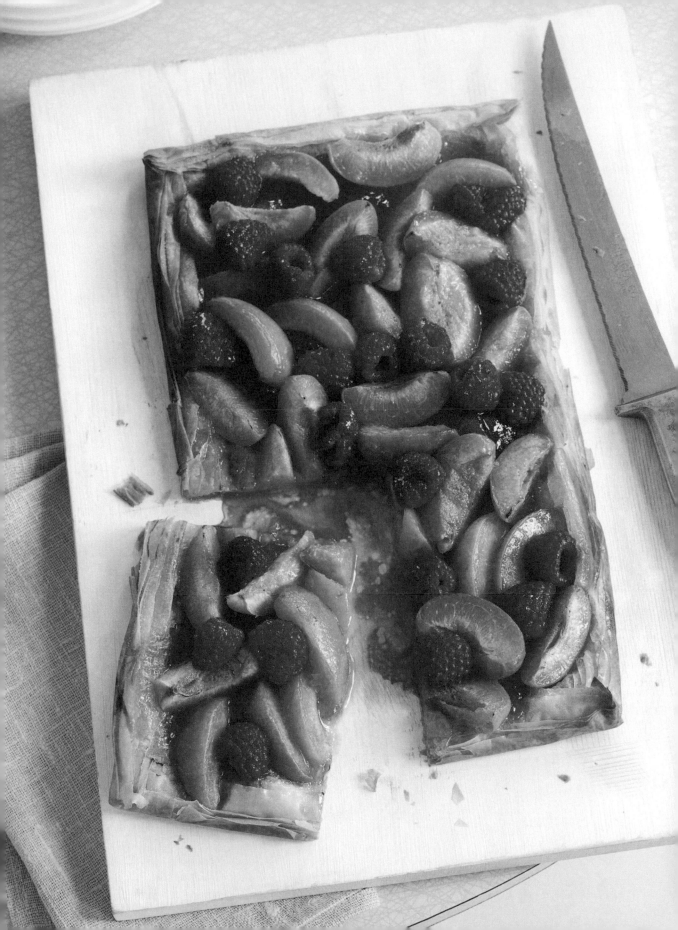

Chocolate & Berry Mousse Pots

A few handfuls of superfruits, such as blueberries, makes each mousse pot 1 of your 5 a day. They also add a little extra sweetness, as there's only 2 teaspoons of added sugar.

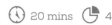 20 mins 4

- 75g/2½oz dark chocolate 70% cocoa solids, grated
- 4 tbsp low-fat yogurt
- 2 large egg whites
- 2 tsp caster sugar
- 350g/12oz berries (try blueberries, raspberries, cherries or a mix)

1 Melt the chocolate in a heatproof bowl over a pan of simmering water, making sure the bowl doesn't directly touch the water. Once melted, allow it to cool for 5–10 mins, then stir in the yogurt.
2 Whisk the egg whites until stiff, then whisk in the sugar and beat until stiff again. Fold the whites into the chocolate mix – loosen the mixture first with a spoonful of egg white, then carefully fold in the rest, keeping as much air as possible.
3 Put the berries into small glasses or ramekins, then divide the mousse on top. Chill in the fridge until set.

PER SERVING 159 kcals, fat 8g, saturates 4g, carbs 19g, sugars 15g, fibre 3g, protein 5g, salt 0.13g

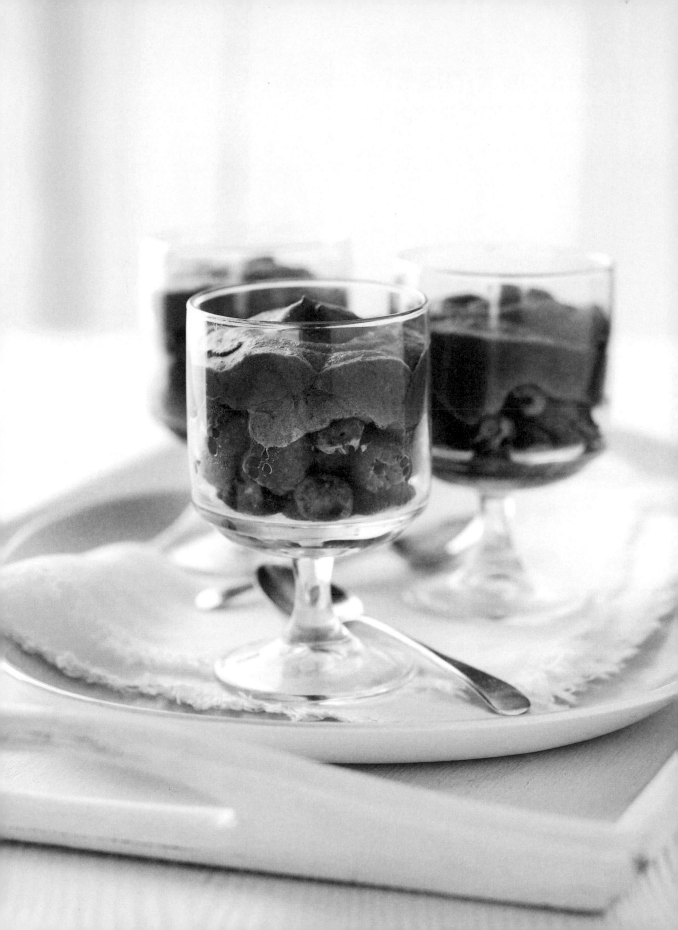

Fromage Frais Mousse with Strawberry Sauce

Making this mousse with cooked meringue as the base means you can happily serve it to vegetarians as there is no need to use gelatine.

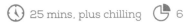 25 mins, plus chilling 6

- 1 large egg white
- 50g/2oz icing sugar, plus 2 tbsp
- grated zest 1 lemon and juice of ½
- 500g tub low-fat fromage frais
- 500g/1lb 2oz strawberries

1 Put the egg white into a heatproof bowl with the icing sugar. Set the bowl over a large pan of simmering water and, using a hand-held electric whisk, whisk for 5 mins until the mixture is light, fluffy and holds peaks when the blades are lifted. Remove from the heat, whisk in the lemon zest, then whisk for a further 2 mins to cool it down.

2 Fold in the fromage frais, then transfer to six glasses or small bowls and chill. Roughly chop half the strawberries and put in the food processor with the 2 tbsp icing sugar and the lemon juice. Whizz to a purée, then press through a sieve to remove the seeds. Chop the remaining strawberries.

3 Spoon the chopped strawberries over the mousses, then spoon a little purée over each. Chill until ready to serve.

PER SERVING 118 kcals, fat none, saturates none, carbs 23g, fibre 1g, sugars 23g, protein 8g, salt 0.13g

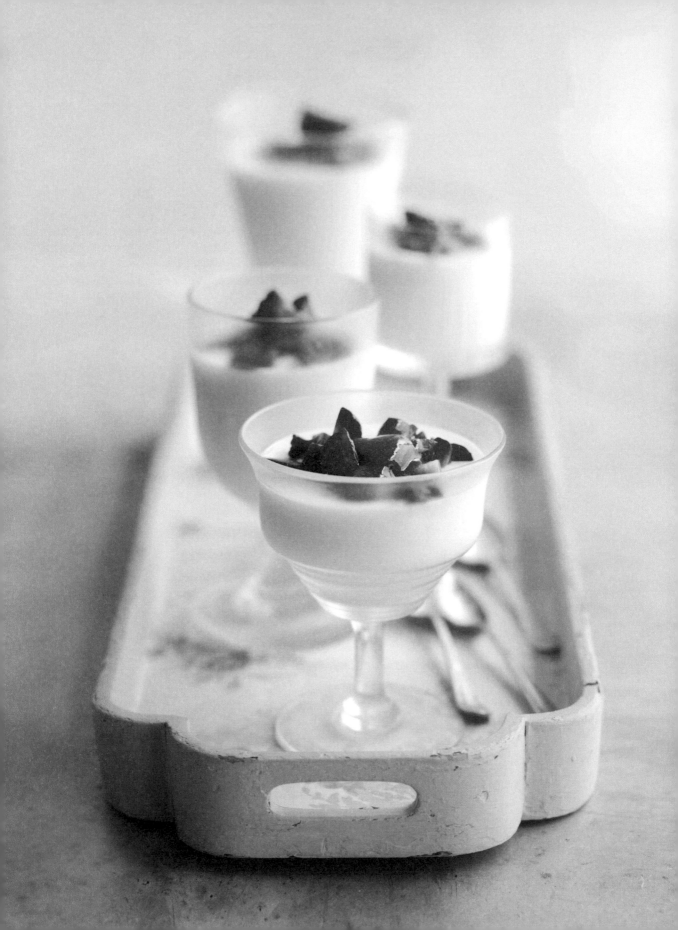

Instant Frozen-berry Yogurt

Craving something sweet after dinner? Keep a bag of mixed berries in your freezer, yogurt in the fridge and this easy pudding is just minutes away.

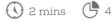 2 mins   4

- 250g/9oz frozen berries, plus extra for serving (optional)
- 250g/9oz fat-free Greek yogurt
- 1 tbsp honey or maple syrup (to taste)

1 Blend the frozen berries, Greek yogurt and syrup or honey in a food processor for 20 seconds, until it forms a smooth ice-cream texture.
2 Scoop into 4 bowls and scatter with extra whole berries to serve, if you like.

PER SERVING 70 kcals, fat none, saturates none, carbs 9g, sugars 9g, fibre 2g, protein 7g, salt 0.1g

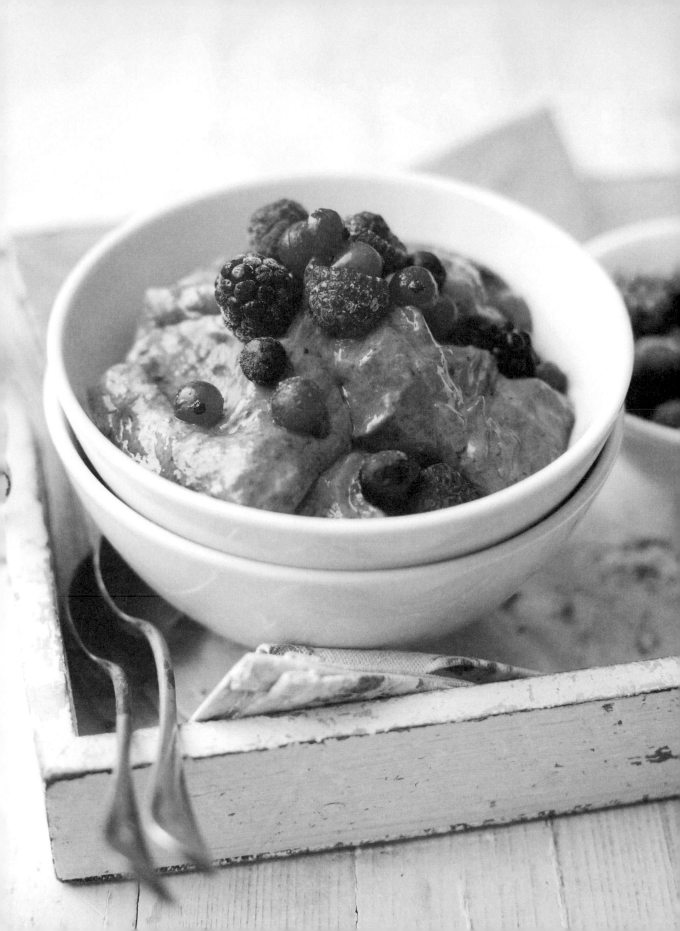

Healthy Banana & Peanut Butter Ice Cream

A speedy ice cream made from ripe, frozen chunks of banana.

🕐 1 hour 10 mins   🍽 4

- 4 ripe bananas, chopped into small chunks, then frozen
- 2 tbsp almond milk or cow's milk
- 1 tbsp peanut butter
- 1 tsp ground cinnamon
- 1 tbsp dark chocolate, grated
- 1 tbsp flaked almonds

1 Tip the frozen bananas and milk into a blender. Blend together to create a smooth consistency. Add the peanut butter and cinnamon, and blend again. Taste and add more cinnamon, if you like.

2 Transfer to a freezerproof container and freeze for 1 hr. Take out of the freezer and serve with grated chocolate and flaked almonds sprinkled over.

PER SERVING 169 kcals, fat 6g, saturates 2g, carbs 24g, sugars 22g, fibre 2g, protein 3g, salt none

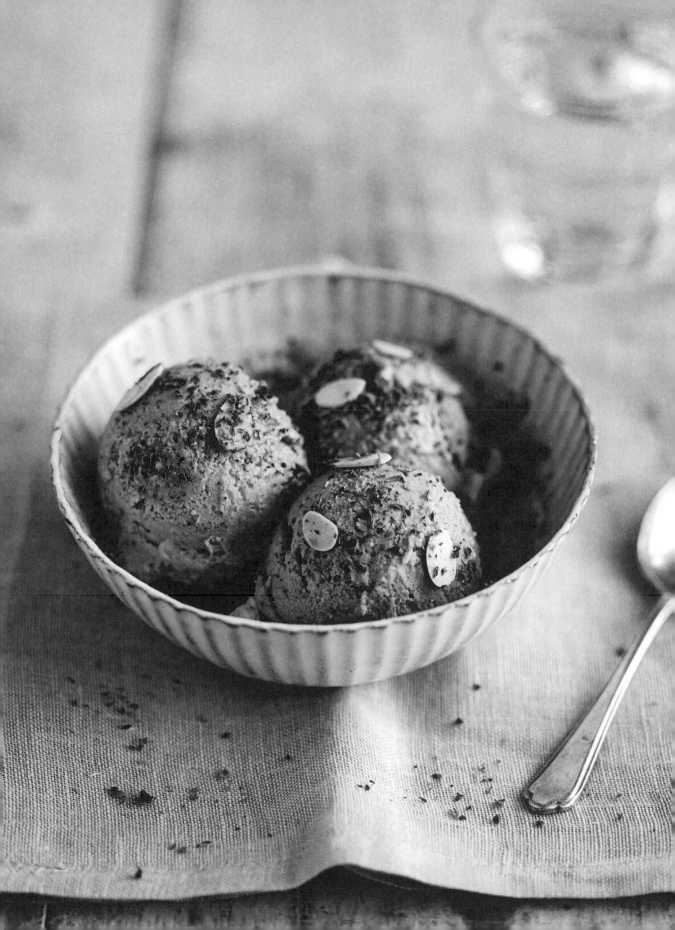

Index